No Matter How Small

No Matter How Small

Understanding Miscarriage and Stillbirth

KRISTEN RIECKE AND PATRICK RIECKE

EMERALD HOPE PUBLISHING HOUSE
FORT WAYNE

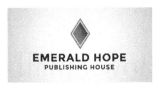

EMERALD HOPE
PUBLISHING HOUSE

Dedication

Stephen Daniel Riecke
10/24/2000

You made us a family.

Though you never came home with us, we miss you always.

Love, Mom, Dad, Daniel, Aidan, Levi, and Kelsey

Contents

About the Authors   ix

Introduction   1

Jayda and Toby's Story   9

1. Statistics Matter   56

2. What If My Loss Was Very Early?   60

3. A Father's Grief   67

4. Faith Matters   70

5. Logistical Matters   76

6. Small Connections: Finding   85
   Community

7. Marker Babies   89

8. Bereaved Mother's Day   92

   Emmaline's Story   94

9. Small Wounds: Insensitive   133
   Comments

10. Honest Emotions   137

11. Support Groups   140

12. Memory-Making in the Hospital   144

13. Compounding Grief   152

14. Funeral for a Stillborn Baby   157

15. Finding Meaning   162

16. Small People Doesn't Mean Small   164
     Grief

     Lori's Story   169

17. Mental Health After Loss   213

18. Why Doesn't My Partner   220
     Understand?

19. Fetal Anomalies   224

20. The Church   227

21. When the Hospital Isn't Hospitable   232

22. Common Threads   235

     In Conclusion   237

     More Resources   240

     Other Books in This Series   244

     Thank You   245

     Acknowledgements   246

About the Authors

Kristen Riecke and her husband Patrick teamed up to bring you this resource on understanding miscarriage and stillbirth. In October 2000, they lost their son, Stephen Daniel, to a second-trimester miscarriage. Since that time they have had the honor of walking alongside hundreds of other loss parents. They blend their voices and years of experience to bring you this resource filled with personal stories and practical advice.

The Riecke family lives in Fort Wayne, Indiana with their four living children. Kristen leads several support groups for loss families and a volunteer program called Kindred Hearts at Parkview Health. She is a self-professed healthy Enneagram 2, an encourager, a connector, and a tender heart. She is also a group fitness instructor at a local YMCA where she has been teaching indoor cycling classes for the last six years. She loves the smell of coffee but can't stand the taste of it and her beverage of choice is Big Red soda. She loves being a football and rugby mom, being the first love of her three teenage boys and "BFF" to her only daughter, Kelsey. She and Patrick have been married over 21 years and she can't wait to see what adventures the next 21 years will bring them.

Kristen and Patrick welcome the opportunity to

share their knowledge and experience with others who might benefit from their work with those who grieve. You can find them at NoMatterHowSmallBook.com and on Facebook & Instagram @NoMatterHowSmallBook.

Patrick is the author of two other books in this series: *How to Talk with Sick, Dying, and Grieving People*, and *How to Find Meaning in Your Life Before it Ends*. He is currently the Director of Chaplaincy and Volunteers, as well as the ethics committee chairperson for Parkview Health. For more content, social media links, to join Patrick's mailing list, or to book Patrick for an event, go to www.PatrickRiecke.com.

Introduction

First of all, we are sorry that you need this book. You probably didn't buy it, borrow it, or download it just because you are curious about the topic. Chances are you have either had a personal experience yourself, like us, or someone close to you has lost a child. We are thankful you found this book, but we wish you didn't need it.

Patrick and I both work with bereaved parents every day, in somewhat different capacities. We've learned more than we could have ever imagined, and the rest of this book is the result of our hearts and experiences.

We want to tell you about those experiences, and about what to expect from this book. But first, we want to tell you about Stephen.

Stephen

Young and in love, we decided it was time to start a family. In no time, I was pregnant.

Patrick was newly employed at a church that we loved. His income was small, but we had good health insurance. Since, at the time, we planned to move overseas for mission work, this seemed like perfect timing. Our baby would be born stateside, accompanied by some of the best medical care in the world. We would be surrounded by family and friends.

To the joy of our parents and families, we announced the news of the pregnancy as soon as we possibly could. Our baby was the first grandchild on my side and one of the last on Patrick's side.

A handful of months later we were at the obstetrician's office for a regular check-up. They tried to detect the baby's heartbeat with a Doppler device but were unsuccessful. We were assured that everything was probably fine, but we were sent to the lobby to wait for an ultrasound. We were so excited at the opportunity to see our little one on the screen again. However, this ultrasound was very different. As soon as the machine was switched on, the silence filled the room. I knew instantly that our lives had changed forever. The tech was unable to find a heartbeat for our son.

The tech was unable to find a heartbeat for our son.

Patrick was just as shocked and sad as I was. We had to make some very difficult decisions. We named our baby Stephen Daniel, after two important men in our lives. I sought support from family and friends who had lost babies. We yelled at God a few times but also felt his comfort and peace.

We collected items for his memory box.

Family and church friends came to see us at our home. Words of sympathy were spoken by many. Hurtful words were spoken by a few.

Sometime later, during a Sunday night prayer service, Patrick spoke about what had happened. He shared in a sermon about how we found comfort in remembering that God also lost a son. Afterward, an elderly couple approached me. Hank and Ginny Vernard. They were the sort of people that we all want to be when we are in our 80s. Sweet, loving, and kind.

Ginny's eyes were wet behind her bifocals when she held my hand.

The words she spoke next have never left us.

"It's been 50 years since we lost our baby. And he still holds a special place in our thoughts and hearts. You never forget."

Our Work

Stephen would be almost nineteen-years-old now. In fact, we have intentionally released this book on his due date as a way to honor his memory. We miss him, and we are thankful for him. His impact didn't stop nineteen years ago.

Ever since my miscarriage, Patrick and I have been connecting with parents having similar experiences–first in church and through personal relationships. Then, Patrick became a staff chaplain at the large hospital about one mile from our home. Little did we know how much that would change our lives.

His team responds to five or six deaths every day, including an average of one miscarriage or stillbirth.

Patrick began responding to patient deaths, including miscarriages and stillbirths, all hours of the day and night. The impact this had on him, and me, could not be overstated. Today, he is the director of the department and leads a large team of chaplains serving ten hospitals twenty-four hours a day. His team responds to five to six deaths every day, including an average of one miscarriage or stillbirth.

Every. Single. Day.

When he started working at the hospital, there was a chaplain who led a small support group for women and men who had experienced pregnancy loss. The chaplain, though well trained, didn't feel particularly equipped to lead the group. Because of this, Patrick came home from work one day and asked if I would be interested in leading the group. Immediately, I said "no". I knew that if I accepted I would need to do it wholeheartedly. That would mean bearing burdens with an unknown number of parents whose arms ached for their children, gone too soon. Besides, our lives were busy with four kids, all home educated at the time, although beginning to transition into public school. Patrick wasn't surprised I declined and has always been a proponent of knowing one's limits. But then he did a very cruel thing. He asked me to pray about it. As soon as I prayed about it, empathy for these unknown parents welled up so significantly I *had* to say yes.

About that time, I met Cori McKenzie, a co-worker who had offered to help with support groups as well. Cori's daughter, Norah, was stillborn a few years earlier. When

> As soon as I prayed about it, empathy for these unknown parents welled up so significantly I *had* to say yes.

she and I met, we quickly discovered we were kindred spirits. She worked in our family birthing center and saw the need to support bereaved moms and dads firsthand. A couple of months later we led the Healing Hearts support group for the first time. Today, we have two more support groups, dozens of connected families, and it just continues to grow.

Most recently, Cori and I had the opportunity to create and coordinate a new volunteer program at our two largest hospitals. The program is called Kindred Hearts. Kindred Hearts volunteers are all specially vetted and trained parents who have had their own miscarriages or stillbirths. They are called in whenever a mom is having a stillborn baby. They companion with her, helping her navigate the shock of the loss, make memories, and helping find the support she needs. It is such an honor to serve these patients and work with these volunteers. The sense of solidarity between these volunteers and patients is sacred. They are *all* a part of a club no one wants to join.

Who is this book for?

This book is for anyone wanting to better understand the experience of miscarriage and stillbirth. Whether your interest is personal or based on a desire to support others, you will benefit greatly. Some of you are in the throes of loss right now. Perhaps you are actively miscarrying or you buried a child very recently. This book *will* help you. It will also help you if your loss was decades ago. On the other hand, if you are a professional (a nurse, physician, chaplain or pastor, counselor, social worker, doula, or midwife), this book will help you empathize and give you a ton of practical advice and education.

The book is set up in three sections. Each section begins with a story of a baby who

The book is set up in three sections.

died. Following each story are brief, candid chapters

about the experience. We wrote those chapters with compassion, but we also wanted to be forthright about the experience, both physically and emotionally. Since we get to see this up close and personal more than most people, we didn't hesitate to be completely honest with you.

Our hearts break with you.

Now, meet our friends, Jayda and Toby...

Jayda and Toby's Story

This was Toby's moment. Jayda would come out of the high school gymnasium doors at any moment. He checked one more time to be sure he didn't still smell from basketball practice. He checked his suit jacket–was it laying just right? He checked the painting–was it facing the right direction?

Check, check, and check.

He inhaled deeply and then exhaled slowly. His hands were cold, and the blood drained out of his face.

Toby first noticed Jayda a couple of years earlier. She walked in with her cheerleading team, wearing her slate gray uniform with green and white trim. Her warm spirit seemed to immediately fill not only Toby's heart but the entire gym. He noticed her, but she didn't seem to notice him. When she did look his way, he could not meet her gaze. Her large eyes, dark and lovely, crowned with striking lashes that fluttered like butterfly wings, were too overwhelming for him.

The next semester, Toby was shocked when he walked into his favorite class, art. Toby was smooth on the basketball court and had good skills. His passing and shooting were quite good, and he had good hands on defense. He was taller than most, and the coach always wanted him to be more aggressive.

However, Toby's parents both knew that *aggressive* was one word that had never described Toby. They used words like *gentle* and *sensitive*. Toby had a big heart. He was quiet, creative, and he loved deeply. That's why art classes were always his favorite. While he had some good skills on the court, he had more skills when he was at the canvas.

Toby was a painter.

But, when he walked into this art class and saw his crush, he felt exposed. The girl he was scared to talk with was in the class where his greatest talents always came to light.

Sure enough, a week later, Jayda noticed Toby in a big way. The students were each recreating a still-life of a vase of daisies. Jayda finished early and was going from classmate to classmate, encouraging their work. Toby felt like she knew everyone's name.

"Nice job, Sam, I like the colors you chose." She could find something kind to say to anyone. Toby thought Sam's painting looked more like spilled lemonade than flowers.

"Wow, Robbie, you made yours really big, I like that."

Suddenly, Toby realized Jayda was coming to him next. He tried not to notice, but he could feel her presence, like a warm glow, standing behind him for nearly a minute. She didn't say anything. Had she walked on by without saying anything to him at all? Finally, Toby turned around, and there she was. Jayda couldn't take her eyes off Toby's canvas.

Her eyes were even bigger than usual and a little glassy. Her mouth was a little agape.

"You ok?" Toby asked, honestly.

When Jayda exhaled, it was obvious something had taken her breath away.

"Toby," she said, as she reached out and touched his elbow. "I had no idea."

Toby looked back at his painting. Then he looked at his feet until he could build the courage to look into the sweetest face he'd ever seen. When he did, he saw a thin trail of a single tear streaking down her curved cheek, her hand still on Toby's arm.

Toby nearly collapsed. He had other paintings he thought were better. He was just having fun with this one. But seeing its effect on Jayda made him feel both free and terrified.

Fortunately, he was saved by the bell. All the students gathered their books. Time for Algebra.

+++

Over time, Jayda and Toby's group of friends started to overlap more and more. That meant they were spending more time around one another. Toby knew that one day he would give that painting to Jayda, the one from their art class together. He hoped she still liked it as much as she did that first day.

So, the painting stood next to him as he waited outside those gym doors. He wore a full blue suit he had borrowed from his dad's closet. He looked like a million dollars, even though only minutes before he was sweaty in his basketball uniform. Toby held a bouquet of daisies in his right hand and a homemade poster in his left hand. The poster had a picture of Jayda, a picture of Toby, and it read, "See Jayda. See Toby. See Jayda and Toby go to the dance together?"

Toby's heart jumped when he saw Jayda emerge from the gym doors with a gaggle of friends. He was nervous enough about how Jayda would react, and he hadn't even thought about so many of her friends being around. He should have because Jayda was never alone. She was a giver and a connector, and that meant she had a million friends.

"Hi Toby," Jayda said before she noticed the sign, the flowers, or the painting. Two or three of her friends had noticed, though. They started whooping and screaming. Toby didn't prepare for the next part. He worked on the sign, carefully picked out the flowers, and repeatedly touched up the painting. But now he might have to talk.

Fortunately, he did not have to say much.

Jayda gave the same look she had given to his canvas in art class, but her lips curled in a huge smile while she raised her hand to her mouth.

"Jayda..." Toby started, although he had no idea what he was going to say.

"Come here, you!" Jayda said and threw her arms around his neck.

By now, the crowd had grown because the girls were screaming. When Jayda hugged Toby, the sign fell to the ground, but yes, everyone could see Toby and Jayda. They could see them not only going to the dance together but could see them spending the rest of their lives together.

+++

While Jayda tried to decide if she liked Toby as more than just a friend, she sought counsel from her mother, as she had many times before. Mom raised Jayda and her two older sisters by herself after their dad left. Mom was patient, hardworking, and wise.

"I don't know, mom. He's so sweet. He's creative and kind. But he's so quiet sometimes, I don't even know what he's thinking," Jayda was vacillating. She felt drawn to Toby, but his personality was so different from hers. She considered nearly everyone her friend, and Toby only had a few close friends. Both of them were church-going kids from families that made faith a priority from the very beginning. Their values were similar but not their personalities.

Jayda and her mom were folding laundry together in the bedroom. Jayda's last phrase "I don't even know what he's thinking" still hung in the air.

Finally, mom spoke. And what she said stuck with Jayda for years to come (all the way through their wedding day).

"Baby girl," Momma said slowly, turning her eyes to Jayda with a look that she recognized.

"There's an old proverb that came to mind the very first time I met Toby. When he made that display for you for the dance, that proverb was confirmed."

She took Jayda's hand to get her attention.

"Jayda," Momma said, "Still waters run deep."

"What does that mean?" Jayda made a puzzled face.

"It means, child, that although everything looks calm and even boring on the outside, that doesn't indicate a lack of depth. That boy kept the painting of the daisies for two years, just because he knew you liked it. A boy that will do that has more to offer than his lack of words. Think about it, Jayda. Toby thought about you every time he looked at that painting for *two years*."

Then she said something that surprised Jayda.

"But," she folded the last shirt and placed it with the others, "he's not *boyfriend* material."

"Wait, what? I thought you liked him?" Jayda was confused.

"I said he's not *boyfriend* material." Momma started for the door, carrying the blue basket, full of folded laundry. "But he *is husband* material," she called back to Jayda, who became quite embarrassed.

"Momma!" She buried her face in the pillows on the bed.

A few years later, the day the young couple would stand before their pastor and exchange marriage vows, Momma had two comments for her sweet, kind, generous daughter.

Jayda was radiant in her wedding dress, the happiest she had ever been in her life. Momma took Jayda's hand and said,

"Still waters run deep..."

"I told you he was husband material."

+++

In the early years of their marriage, Jayda worked at a diner as a waitress. She was every customer's favorite. She couldn't remember their regular order, but she always remembered their names, their stories, families, good times, and hard days.

It wasn't unusual to see her chatting with a customer a little too long, giving some good advice, a listening ear, and then following up with them a week later to see how things were going. Her tips were hefty because people didn't just like her–they loved her because she loved them, and made them feel special, even if they regularly had to remind her to bring the side of fries they ordered.

Toby happened into a job as a mail carrier. He liked the job just fine. It was quiet and purposeful and gave him time to think, time to plan his next painting, or date nights with Jayda. Toby had two loves–Jayda and his art. However, a third love was in Toby's future–his near future.

Toby walked the same mail route for his first two years as a mailman. He liked the predictability. Well, the route was mostly predictable. Then there was Jean.

Jean was an older woman, a widow, who always seemed to be watching for Toby to come by. Sometimes she had a bottle of water for him, but usually, she had a job for which she wanted his help.

Once, she had a broom in her hand and was trying to clean her little porch.

"Toby, can you help me? I can't reach the top corners."

"Sure, Auntie Jean." She insisted for months that Toby call her that. He finally gave in.

Another time it was a jar lid that she could not get loose. Then a nail she needed to be driven in so she could hang a new frame.

It wasn't usually much. When Toby mentioned the little jobs to Jayda, she'd say, "Auntie Jean just needs a friend."

One day, Toby was bracing for Auntie Jean's daily request as he reached her house, but she was nowhere in sight. Her front door was open slightly. Toby brought her mail up to the porch and called out, quietly at first, "Auntie Jean?" Then a little louder, "Auntie Jean!"

It was strange. She didn't drive, and she was almost always waiting for him. He stood at the front door, looking through the opening, but could not see a thing. Although his boss would not approve of him going into the home of a customer uninvited, Toby took a deep breath and drew upon his deep waters. He could tell something was wrong. Gently, he pushed the door to Auntie Jean's house open, calling her name all the while.

Just two steps into her entryway, he saw Auntie Jean's feet, sticking out from the living room where she was lying on her side.

"Auntie Jean!" Toby yelled.

She looked up at him but said nothing. Her coffee had spilled on the white carpet. It was still warm when he knelt next to her. He pulled out his phone. He stayed with her until the medics arrived and whisked her away to the hospital.

The next day, Jayda had a card and flowers ready when Toby got home from work, and they headed to the hospital to see Auntie Jean. As soon as they stepped into the room, Auntie Jean called out in a loud voice, "My hero!" Toby was embarrassed.

Auntie Jean and a nurse explained that the stroke must have happened just a few minutes before Toby came to deliver the mail.

"Time is critical when it comes to stroke care," the nurse told Toby as Jayda squeezed his arm. "If you hadn't stopped... if you hadn't called for an ambulance..." She looked at Jean.

"I'd be dead!" Auntie Jean called out loudly, then cackled. She joked that if she was gone that Toby could get home to his lovely wife a little earlier.

Shortly thereafter, Toby's route changed, but he and Jayda continued to stop by Auntie Jean's house now and then to help out.

+++

The young couple wasn't exactly trying to get pregnant when they did. Sitting in their bedroom, they were supposed to wait five minutes before reading the test. But Toby could not wait.

"Stop!" Jayda smiled. "It's only been two minutes!"

"I'm checking again," Toby said after another thirty seconds had passed. His still waters were rippling slightly.

Jayda was trying to be nonchalant, putting some clothes away in the bedroom when she heard a loud whoop in the bathroom, followed by Toby's long hands clapping together with a sudden force.

She could barely turn around before his tall frame came flooding into the room, knees crouched and arms spread wide. He scooped Jayda up, his forearms just under her backside, and his face right at her belly.

"We're going to have a baby! Baby, baby, baby!" Toby was giddy with laughter and joy and was mentally composing one painting after another for his precious daughter (he just knew it was a girl).

"What? Put me down, Toby!" Jayda laughed as she playfully smacked his shoulders.

When she rushed into the bathroom, what she saw confirmed Toby's exclamation. She fell into his arms and cried and prayed. At that moment, for Jayda, crying and praying were the same thing.

"Congratulations, Momma," Toby said to Jayda.

"Congratulations, Daddy," Jayda said to Toby.

As Toby bent over to kiss Jayda, her long lashes flashed up at him, and Toby wondered, *What am I going to do with a second pair of lashes like this under my roof?*

+++

The pastor who performed their wedding, Pastor Thomas, was a little younger than Toby's dad and had been a constant source of support for Toby. He understood Toby's quiet way, even though he was more gregarious himself. So, it wasn't unusual that Pastor Thomas's phone lit up once Toby and Jayda told their families about their surprise news.

"Pastor?" Toby's voice was bright.

"Hey, Toby, how you doin'?" Pastor Thomas was proud of Toby. He was a good man and cared deeply for his wife and the church. Jayda was an important part of the church, as well. Upon Pastor Thomas's request, she had just started a new ministry. The ministry was for young moms who needed a little help. She coordinated baby showers, met with the moms to give them friendship and resources, and prayed for them.

"I'm doing great, Pastor. I've got something to tell you." Toby wasn't one to beat around the bush.

"What's the word, Toby? I hope you haven't had to play hero again for anyone on your mail route." Pastor Thomas loved to tell the story about Toby and Auntie Jean.

"No, nothing like that, Pastor. It's about Jade. And

me. We're... pregnant!" The words bubbled out of his heart.

"Oh my goodness, Toby, are you serious? That's so great! I'm so happy for you. Praise the Lord, this is a reason to give God thanks and praise, indeed." Pastor Thomas replied. "You two are doing it, right, Toby. You and Jayda are faithful young people. You're an example for others to follow. It's no surprise God wants to give you a blessing like this." Then he said something Toby would remember later. "You two deserve it."

"Thanks, Pastor," Toby was thankful for Pastor Thomas, and before they ended the call, Pastor Thomas had a request.

"Say, Tobias," that wasn't actually Toby's name, but Pastor liked to call him that. "I was going to tell Jayda this Sunday, but we've got another ministry opportunity. I just learned that there is another young lady in need of her ministry. She's the niece of a woman at church. She just found out that she's pregnant, too. But it's not such a happy situation, Toby. I'm not sure she will keep the pregnancy, and she's not sure who the dad is. She's broke and just lost her job. Things with her folks are rocky. She's gonna need a lot of support. I think God knew what he was doing when he had both of these women conceive at the same time. Jayda can be a special blessing to her."

"Ok, Pastor, I'll let Jayda know." But Toby was a little uneasy about it. He knew that Jayda had a lot on her plate—work, her pregnancy, and she was already working with a few other mothers. He wondered if Pastor Thomas was right about it being a good thing that they were pregnant at the same time. He could imagine it being very difficult for both of them. Comparisons would be inevitable. Toby trusted Pastor, but later he remembered this uneasy feeling.

That Sunday, Jayda met the young lady Pastor had described. It was clear she was in a world of hurt. She dominated the conversation with Jayda, mostly telling her how upset she was to be pregnant. She had a two-year-old son already, and from what Jayda picked up, his dad wasn't worth too much. This young lady wasn't sure what she was going to do next.

Jayda, as always, went into action to help. She set up temporary housing for her, got her enrolled in some programs to be sure she had food and other necessities. She scheduled a special baby shower for a few months down the road, and let all the other women at church know when and where they should be to bless this needy woman and her two children.

All the while, Toby was thinking constantly about their baby, their *daughter*, according to him. It was still early in the pregnancy, but he had already picked out his favorite name for a little girl.

+++

There are some occurrences for which one cannot prepare.

For example, a healthy, bright, faith-filled, fully in love couple should be able to expect to welcome their first child without any significant problems.

However, at one of Jayda's early appointments for the baby, something happened for which they were totally unprepared.

They were excited to see their baby on an ultrasound for the first time. They had heard the heartbeat (*her* heartbeat according to Toby), but now they would be able to see her tiny face and body. In the lobby, the young couple held hands and exchanged excited glances. Jayda let out little giggles of anticipation.

But when they reached the room where the ultrasound would happen, it was dark and cold. Jayda lay on the table. This time, she had a feeling; a sense that something was wrong.

Toby was still oblivious as the technician was silent, and so was the machine. Slowly tears started to form in the corners of Jayda's lovely dark eyes. She blinked her big eyelashes.

Finally, Jayda spoke.

"There's no heartbeat, is there?"

Toby felt a little like he did that day outside the gymnasium doors, but this time for a very different reason. All the blood drained out of his face and his hands were instantly cold and sweaty. His mind was racing.

They fumbled through the rest of the appointment. The doctor said the baby had simply died at some point before they came to the office. That much they knew already. They learned that if Jayda didn't miscarry on her own, she might have to have surgery. Jayda had never had surgery before. It made her feel a little scared.

Back in the parking lot, the couple closed the car doors and just sat still for a moment, totally blindsided. It was the first cool day of fall. Leaves started to fall around the car. The sky was gray. The clouds were an unmoving ceiling in the heavens.

The car was so quiet. Toby didn't start the ignition, and no one else was around.

Jayda was full-on sobbing now. Toby followed suit.

He was super sad about the baby, but watching Jayda cry as she had never cried before broke his heart, too.

"We never even asked if it really was a girl..." Toby said.

"It was probably too early to tell anyway, baby." Jayda's answer didn't make either of them feel any better.

"Is it okay if we think of the baby as a girl, even though we don't know for sure?" Toby asked.

Now Jayda recognized how sad Toby was and how much she wanted to put a little girl, his little girl, into his arms–how much she wanted to watch him love a little girl with the deep waters in his heart just the way he loved her. Now, all those hopes and dreams were gone. In a moment.

"I think I'd like that, sweetie," Jayda said. "What about a name?"

"I have one in mind," Toby said. Jayda wasn't surprised that he'd already been thinking about it. "What about Amani? It means *faith*."

Now that Jayda's little girl had a name, which she loved, she felt even sadder. She was happy Amani had a name, but it made the miscarriage feel so much more real. She hadn't lost a faceless, nameless, possibility. She felt like she lost... a daughter.

And, of course, she had.

Amani died, and Toby and Jayda would never be the same.

+++

A few days later Toby found himself in the waiting room at the surgery center.

Although they hadn't been trying to get pregnant, Toby was so happy with the thought of their little girl, Amani, becoming a part of their lives.

Little clothes.

Little cries.

Big eyes with long eyelashes looking up at him.

It all seemed so perfect.

Until Amani died.

Even after lots of tears over the past few days, Toby was still in shock. He was angry and sad, and mostly confused. After all, Pastor Thomas had said it. He and Jayda deserved to have this blessing. They were doing things the right way. God had blessed them with a child. Had God taken Amani away? Pastor Thomas seemed to think so.

"God needed another angel in heaven," Pastor said when he heard the news. He told them that God must have needed Amani more than they did.

While Pastor had good intentions, these comments stung. Jayda and Toby always thought God was loving and generous. Now Pastor Thomas seemed to be telling them that God took away their innocent child. It seemed so cruel.

After Jayda went into surgery, Jayda's mom and sisters walked down the hall to get coffee. Pastor Thomas and Toby's dad sat with Toby in the lobby. Toby's dad was comfortable with the silence that fell on them when the ladies left, but Pastor Thomas shifted in his seat. Small talk doesn't go very far on days like these, and even pastors can struggle to find the right words to say.

Toby's head was buried in his hands, his elbows on his knees. He was feeling a new emotion now: fear. Thinking of Jayda being in surgery, he began to panic about her safety. Sure, the doctor said this was a quick and simple procedure, but what if Jayda was allergic to the medicine? Or she had problems breathing? What if she got sick while she was waking up?

His weary mind, so full of feelings for Jayda and

Amani, the loves of his life, was spinning out of control.

Unfortunately, that's when Pastor Thomas broke the silence.

"Toby," he said. "I just can't help but think God's got a reason for all this. I know you are hurting now, brother, but just you wait. God works all things for our good when we put our trust in him." Toby's dad shot a sidelong look at Pastor Thomas, who did not get the hint. "God never gives us more than we can handle, son. Can't you see it?"

What Toby's dad could see was that his son was losing control. Sensitive Toby's breathing became heavy, like a bull about to charge. All those still waters inside of Toby were becoming a tsunami. His jaw clenched and his eyes were on fire. He was sad. He was angry. He was afraid.

Then, Toby's dad stood.

He was a tall man with a thin frame, not unlike Toby's. Silver ringed the edge of his hairline and faded into solid black at the crown of his head. He dressed up every day. The day his daughter-in-law had to say goodbye to his granddaughter was no exception. His button-down shirt was blue and checked with thin white stripes. His slacks, neatly pressed, were a light tan while his corduroy sports jacket was dark brown. He removed his cap before he addressed Pastor Thomas, who was still seated. He was angry, like Toby, but his words were measured.

"Pastor, this ain't Sunday, and it's not the time for a sermon. After all, did Jesus preach at the widow in the gospels when her son died? Did Jesus preach at Martha when her brother died? Wasn't Abraham allowed to mourn his wife for as long as he wished? And King David, Pastor. You ought to know about King David. King David's child was so sick, and then he died. Did David not mourn for his son, Pastor? Did he not collapse in tears and go without food for days? And yet, he was a man after God's own heart, as you know, Pastor Thomas. You do know about King David, don't you, Pastor?" Others in the lobby started to stare.

Pastor Thomas's mouth was wide open, and Toby's eyes were wide open. Toby never heard his dad speak with anything but respect to Pastor Thomas. His dad's tone wasn't mean, but he *was* indignant. The last time Toby heard his dad sound like this was when he accidentally scratched one of his dad's favorite records when he was in fifth grade.

As his dad spoke, Toby's anger melted a bit, and his jaw relaxed.

His dad continued. "And don't you remember Job? Do you remember the saddest part of all the troubles that came upon Job, Pastor Thomas?" At the next phrase, his voice began to shake. "His children, pastor. His children. All of them..." now his tears flowed in rivulets down his creased cheeks. "Dead. Every last one of them. Job didn't need no sermon, Pastor, and neither does Toby. Job needed friends. He needed friends to sit down, shut up, and cry. Now Pastor," Toby's dad's furry eyebrows raised, as did his pointer finger on his lifted hand, "that is precisely what we are going to do today. You are welcome to stay if you can do that. If you can sit here, be quiet, and mourn with us over Amani, we would be honored to count you as one of our friends."

Toby had always loved his dad.

Now he loved him more.

+++

Later that evening, Jayda's mom arrived with a slow cooker full of chicken and noodles, a large crock of buttery mashed potatoes, two dozen yeast rolls, green beans with little pieces of bacon mixed in, and two pecan pies.

Jayda's sisters and Toby's parents arrived a few minutes later and they all sat down in the couple's tiny kitchen. Their table only had four chairs, so three more were collected from the family room and everyone squeezed together. The house was full of the sounds and smells of the best kind of love; love mixed with tears and laughter.

"I heard you preached at Pastor Thomas..." Jayda's oldest sister prodded Toby's dad.

"Hmm?" Toby's dad replied.

Jayda chimed in since she had only heard part of the story. "Yeah, Dad, what got you so riled up?"

He was eating pecan pie as his appetizer.

"Oh, it's always been a hard pill for me to swallow.

Some people think you gotta cheer people up when they're sad. As though God didn't give us the ability to grieve. You guys lost a baby. A baby! You lost hopes, dreams, plans, expectations. You were stopped in your tracks." As he said this, Toby's dad raised both hands, palms facing out. "You were picking out Amani's name, getting her room ready, shopping for clothes, and praying for her every night. I don't doubt that there is a purpose for Amani's life. But I can't handle people telling me there's any good reason for her death. She's an innocent child. Your child. My grandbaby."

He could have gone on, and every woman in the room hoped he would, but he'd said his piece.

After dinner, Jayda's sisters helped clean up while she and her mom settled into the pink love seat in their front room. The late evening sun was fading and the shadow of autumn leaves danced through the large front window.

"Tell me how you're feeling after surgery, baby." Mom reached out and took Jayda's hand.

"Not bad. I'm tired, and I'm sad."

"Of course you are, sweetheart. I know how happy you were when you found out you were expecting. Almost as happy as Toby!" They laughed together.

"Will I ever feel normal again, Mom?" To her mom, Jayda's sweet face looked like a child again.

"Not exactly..." Mom paused and took a breath. Jayda knew her mom had a miscarriage after her middle sister before Jayda was born, but mom hadn't mentioned it since Jayda found out Amani died.

"I keep thinking that I know how you feel." Mom paused and looked directly into Jayda's eyes. "But that's not fair. You're not me. And this isn't my miscarriage. I don't want to shift our conversation to my experience. I want to support you. This isn't about me."

"Well," Jayda asked softly, "Do you mind telling me about your miscarriage?"

Mom grinned a little grin and started, "I've always imagined that baby was my son..." For the next two hours, they swapped stories, not to compare, but to connect.

+++

The following week Jayda went back to work at the diner and Toby was back on his mail route. Toby was glad to be back to work. Jayda thought she would be glad.

So many of her customers were regulars, that everyone wanted to know how her pregnancy was going. It was impossible to avoid questions. Each time she saw a new person come through the door, she became anxious.

Did he know I was pregnant? She would think. *Will she ask me how the baby is doing, or comment on the pregnancy?*

Sometimes they did, and sometimes they didn't. Both experiences were hard. She wanted Amani's life to be recognized and honored. But she also didn't want to have to talk about her grief while she was refilling cups of coffee or bringing a dessert menu.

"How's our little mommy doing?" an older gentleman asked, innocently enough. He sat at the counter by himself.

"Hanging in there," she said, hoping that would be enough to satisfy him.

It wasn't.

"When's the little one due?" She should have been ready for such a natural question, but she wasn't. She felt backed into a corner, and she had only been back to work for an hour.

"Well," she started, not sure where she was going. "Well, actually, I miscarried last week." She felt like she was admitting to a crime.

"Oh no." He barely looked up from his coffee. "Well, thank God you're young. You'll have another one," he said before placing his order.

Jayda felt like boiling water had been dumped on her head. Her cheeks were hot, and her hands started to shake.

This was going to be even harder than she thought.

Of course, her co-workers knew what had happened since she took a few days off work.

"I had a miscarriage when I was about your age," said an older woman who worked at the grill in the kitchen. "But we women just gotta soldier on. I didn't even miss a day of work."

Jayda felt like she had stepped out of the frying pan and into the fire. She wondered if everyone at work resented her for taking a few days off to mourn for Amani.

"Well, I had surgery," Jayda knew she shouldn't have to provide a reason for missing work after the death of a family member, but she tried to anyhow.

Over the next week, Jayda had to explain to more than a dozen regular customers that her pregnancy had ended suddenly. She heard a lot of comments from well-meaning people that stuck with her.

"Time heals all wounds," said one sweet old lady. That almost felt true.

"You've got to move on, sweetie. These things happen," said another customer. Jayda cried during her break. Last week, she was a train traveling full steam ahead to motherhood. Amani's death totally derailed her. Now she was just supposed to *move on*?

Nearly everyone wanted to know if they planned to try again. That was an easy one to answer; of course. But whenever she thought about another pregnancy, fear arose in her heart over the possibility of having another loss.

With Toby's help, she was ready whenever someone said "everything happens for a reason." Jayda did believe that God had her best interests in mind, even after Amani died. But she would not allow this comment to belittle their grief. So, she had a prepared response, and Toby helped her practice the reply.

Whenever she heard anything like *everything happens for a reason* she decided to say, "That's true. But when we're in the middle of the storm, it's hard to see the rainbow."

She and Toby stood in their little bedroom, just outside the bathroom door where Toby had impatiently read the positive pregnancy test. She asked him to pretend to be a customer and tell her that everything happens for a reason. Then she was supposed to say her line: *That's true. But when you're in the middle of the storm, it's hard to see the rainbow.* On her first try, her mind dissolved into a fog of feelings about God, questions she had about the future, and thoughts about Amani. However, after a few attempts, Jayda could even grin a little at the end of her simple proclamation.

The next day, when a woman told her that everything happens for a reason, Jayda was ready. She'd already used her response several times, and it was working. It was protecting her heart and giving her a way to respond to this accidentally hurtful comment. But this woman surprised her.

Jayda was waiting to take her order at the counter when the conversation came up.

"I didn't see you when I came for lunch last week. Were you on vacation? You deserve it, that's for sure." The woman was glancing between her menu and Jayda's sweet face.

"I wish," Jayda said. She knew the woman wouldn't settle for that reply.

"Were you sick? Everything okay?"

"No, everything's not okay. I lost my pregnancy last week."

After a few more exchanges, the woman looked back at her menu and said, "Well, you know what they say. Everything happens for a reason."

"That's true," Jayda said, her new lines bubbling up, "But when you're in the middle of the storm, it's hard to see the rainbow."

The woman put her menu down. She looked at Jayda with an expression that Jayda could not quite interpret. When she blinked, Jayda could tell her eyelids were holding back tears.

"You right about that, Jayda. You right about that."

Jayda put her notepad down and walked around the counter. The woman opened her arms and Jayda squeezed her tight for a good two minutes. Neither one of them said anything more.

+++

That night, back at the house, Jayda told Toby about the woman.

"What do you think that was about?" He asked.

"I sure don't know. But I think more people are hurting out there than I ever realized, Toby. I think that being honest about my grief helped that woman today."

"That's so great, Jade," Toby said. "What's been the worst thing that someone said?" Jayda had worked the better part of two weeks, so he wondered if there was one comment that she was holding on to more than others.

Jayda shuddered a bit as she picked at her dinner. She set her fork down and picked up her drink. Toby heard her sniffle.

"I'm embarrassed to say so, but it was a comment about my faith." Toby's elbows were on the table and his long arms stretched across so far he could almost reach Jayda.

"Well, one guy told me I just needed to have faith. That I needed to trust God." Toby had to admit it didn't seem like the harshest comment.

"What made that hurt so much?" He could feel her pain, as he always could.

"Because, Toby," Jayda shouted. "What the heck do you think I am trying to do? Every morning I wake up without a baby inside me, I pray to God to help me trust him. To help me have faith. To help me believe that he's really there and that he really loves me. I pray that he helps me understand why Amani died. I'm trying harder than ever to have faith in God."

Toby came across the room and wrapped his arms around Jayda.

He prayed. When he prayed he yelled a little. He remembered Pastor Thomas saying that people of faith sometimes yell at God. So, he knew God would understand.

After he finished, he looked Jayda in the eyes, and

with a very serious voice, he said, "If anyone else ever says that to you, just call me. I'll punch him right in the nose."

The thought of gentle big-hearted Toby punching someone made Jayda laugh out loud.

Toby still had the other mom at church on his mind.

"Jade, I've been thinking." Toby was always thinking. "About the mom at church that Pastor Thomas wanted you to care for. The one who's also pregnant." Toby realized that Jayda wasn't pregnant anymore, but he didn't correct himself. "I didn't have a great feeling about it, to begin with. And now..."

"Her baby will be Amani's *marker baby*." Jayda was also thinking.

"Amani's what?" Toby asked.

"Amani's marker baby. That means that whenever we see her baby, we will think about Amani and how she would be the same age; that she would be doing that thing; crawling, walking, going to school, you know." Jayda explained.

"Yeah, well, that's going to be heavy," was all he could say. "I don't think you can, I mean, I don't think you should..."

"I know Tobias." Jayda playfully called him by the name Pastor Thomas used for him. "But I'll be okay. She needs someone like me to lift her up, to encourage her. I can do it."

Jayda's heart was in the right place like it always was, but she was wrong.

She couldn't do it.

+++

Auntie Jean called her 'hero' and asked if he could stop by to help her with a couple of little jobs around her house. So, Toby stopped by after work the next day. He just knew Auntie Jean would take it hard when she found out that they lost the baby, but he had to tell her.

"How's your little lady doing, Toby? I bet her belly's getting big by now."

"Actually it's not," Toby was a bit of a slow talker normally, but especially when he had hard news. That's why it was easy for Auntie Jean to jump in.

"Oh don't worry about that, she'll be huge before you know it," Auntie Jean said before turning to head into the kitchen.

"Actually, she won't." Toby was bracing for how upset Auntie Jean would become.

"Auntie, Jayda miscarried a couple of weeks ago." He stood tall in her foyer, his head cocked to one side, sorry he had to deliver such horrible news.

But Auntie Jean's response haunted Toby for months.

Dressed in her long multi-colored housecoat, she waved her right hand as she turned to enter the kitchen. "Well, at least you didn't have time to get too attached."

Toby was too stunned for words. *Unattached* was the least appropriate description of how he felt about Amani. He numbly completed the tasks Auntie

Jean had on her list and went home. He didn't tell Jayda. The only reason he didn't was that he couldn't.

+++

Over the next few weeks, each time Jayda interacted with the other mom from church, she tried to grin and bear it. She didn't want to admit it, but just thinking about her gave Jayda anxiety and a little anger. Jayda was never angry before Amani died. So, some of these feelings were new, and she wasn't sure how to handle them.

She tried to ignore them.

"How's it going with your new pupil?" Pastor Thomas bellowed down the hall one Sunday.

"Great," Jayda lied. "We've been meeting on Tuesday nights. Her new place is working out well, and I think she's staying clean."

"Praise the Lord. Thank you for investing in her, Jayda." Then Pastor Thomas let his preacher voice fade. "Jayda, I'm so sorry about your baby."

"Me too, Pastor. Me too."

It was the first signal that deep inside Pastor's heart, he was still listening to the sermon Toby's dad gave him in that lobby last fall. Pastors don't always know how to react when they come face-to-face with people's most difficult moments. Especially if those moments feel like they go against the message they preach. But Pastor Thomas loved this family. So, he was going to figure it out. He just needed a little more time.

+++

Jayda's mom visited her for lunch before Jayda went to work on a cold January day. Mom made thick-sliced turkey sandwiches and served them with leftover seven-layer salad. Jayda made it through the holidays. It was a little like groping in the dark. The regular joys of the season felt different. Jayda was still herself, just sad. She could see why some women would be truly depressed. She knew it could be worse, but she was still sad.

She did even more supporting of the pregnant woman at church through the holidays, with the baby shower just around the corner. Jayda hated to admit it, but Toby was right. It was proving to be a real struggle for her. Every time she saw this woman, she was more resentful.

Mom knew it, too.

"How's it going mentoring your friend from church?" Mom asked without emotion.

"She's *not* my friend, mom." Jayda's anger made her mom set her glass down on the table. "She's just one of the moms Pastor wants me to help, that's all. And it's fine. She's doing just fine. Her baby's doing just fine–growing right on schedule, of course."

Mom wasn't pushy. But she was keenly observant, and she noticed that last phrase.

"Of course, huh?"

"Yep, even though she was on drugs and drinking all the time when she got pregnant. Even though she has no idea which guy is the dad. Even though

I'm not sure she even really wants the baby, everything is going," Jayda wadded up her linen napkin, clenched her teeth, and said, "*just fine.*"

"Hmm. Well, that's good, right?" Mom asked, simply, even though it was clear that it was not okay with Jayda.

"Of course it's good. But doesn't it seem just a little ironic? Just a tad unfair?" She was asking a woman who knew the pain of miscarriage as well.

Then Jayda's real feelings came to the surface.

"I mean why would God...?" she could not bring herself to finish the question. "Why would God...?"

"Sweetie," mom came around the table, took the wadded up napkin, and slid her left arm over her baby's shoulder. It had been months since Amani had died, but Jayda's body convulsed with grief in her work uniform.

"Sweetie, there are no words that will explain why this happened. No explanation will ever be enough to lessen your sadness about Amani even one iota. Your tears. Your anger. They are *right*. That's because it hurts. And I wish I could tell you that it'll all go away. But I owe it to you to be honest with you, just like you have been honest with me. Even all these years later, I am still sad, still angry, about the baby I lost. Even last week, I thought to myself that if your big brother was still alive, that maybe he would help. That he would be so caring, so loving, a little like your Toby, and I miss him something awful. I know that sounds silly because I never even laid my eyes on him, but I do. I miss him. I miss Amani. And I love you, sweetie."

Mom had not even tried to answer Jayda's deep question about why God let this happen. But somehow, when Jayda went to work that afternoon, she felt more comforted than she had in some time.

+++

That night after her shift, Jayda and Toby sat in their little kitchen for a late dinner, as they often did. Jayda told Toby about her mom's question.

"I hate to admit it when you're right, Toby," she grinned at her best friend. "But I can't keep helping that mom from church. She needs help. And she deserves it. But it's not doing either of us any good. It's just making me more mad and jealous every time I think about her."

Toby knew this was hard for Jayda. She wanted to help and serve everyone. It was one of her best attributes. So, drawing a boundary like this wasn't easy.

Toby was the thinker of the two, but Jayda was intuitive. She could tell there was something Toby hadn't told her about how he was handling his grief.

She knew better than to prod and push if Toby wasn't ready. So she pulled out the packet of information the doctor's office had given them after the miscarriage. She removed a pamphlet on local grief counselors.

Toby was carrying his tension in his shoulders. He still wasn't sure how to interact with Pastor Thomas at church. He was still carrying Auntie Jean's comment with him like a lead weight around his neck. He missed Amani something awful.

"Looks like this one doesn't even charge," Jayda was selecting a counselor without asking Toby.

"This one what?" Toby asked.

"Oh, I realized after my talk with mom today that we need to get into some counseling. You know, not that anything is wrong with us, but to help us grieve well if a person can even do such a thing."

Toby hadn't painted since Amani's death. When Jayda talked about being stuck in grief, grieving well, and finding a counselor, for some reason, the fact that he had not painted in months rushed to his mind.

He just couldn't paint right now. Painting had brought him so much joy since he was a little boy, but now the colors were all dull. He wondered if Jayda had noticed. Of course, she had. That was one of the main reasons she was selecting a counselor for them. Toby made it a practice to not question Jayda. He continued that practice, and about a week later the two of them sat in an office with a professional counselor.

+++

The winter was long, but the counselor helped Jayda and Toby grieve well. They did memory-making activities. They made a Christmas ornament with Amani's name, even though Christmas had already passed. They finished a baby book for her with all their memories. They framed their favorite picture from Amani's pregnancy. In the photo Jayda wore a sundress, her sweet face glowing, with Toby standing right behind her, wrapping his arms around her. They put the frame in the middle of their front room with the big windows, where every visitor could see it.

Jayda quickly gained more boldness when she talked with other women about her miscarriage. It was hard to believe how common the experience was. Nearly every woman at church had either miscarried themselves or knew a woman who had.

Jayda posted thoughts about miscarriage and its unique pain online, had coffee with other moms to talk about it, and started praying for more opportunities to help women in this position.

In April, Toby and Jayda's counselor asked how they were going to celebrate Mother's Day.

"By trying to pretend it doesn't exist," Jayda said. She gave a wry grin.

Their rapport with the counselor had grown significantly, and they all laughed.

The counselor had an idea, "What if you organized a little event for Bereaved Mother's Day? It's the Sunday before Mother's Day, and could be a good time to get a group of ladies together who have lost babies."

"I love that," Jayda was finding a new outlet for her innate desire to care for other people. Her gaze shot at Toby. "What do you say, babe? Remember that time we got our friends together and you helped us each create a simple painting? What if we did that for moms, and you picked a painting that could hold meaning for us in our grief?" Jayda planned the whole event instantly.

Toby rubbed the back of his head and tried to look away. "I don't know if you noticed, Jade, but I haven't painted since Amani died."

"Is that right?" The counselor replied. "Tell me about that."

Toby mumbled some lame reasons why he wasn't painting, but in his mind, he just kept seeing Auntie Jean as she waved her hand and said, "Well, at least you didn't have enough time to get attached." So, he finally told Jayda, and their counselor, the whole story. Auntie Jean's comment held so much power for the past few months. He felt like something was wrong with him for feeling so attached to Amani. But when he said it out loud, he realized that while it was hurtful, it was also ridiculous.

"She doesn't know you very well, does she, Toby?" A deep thinker and feeler like Toby was like an open book to a counselor.

Toby wiped a tear. "I don't suppose she does."

The counselor gave them an assignment.

"By this time next week, Jayda, I want you to make a list of the moms you will invite for Bereaved Mother's Day. Toby, I want you to think of three designs for paintings you could lead the group through."

Toby swallowed hard and asked his question. "So it's okay that I still feel so attached to Amani?"

The counselor's answer was straightforward.

"Toby, Amani is your daughter. Your only child. Your sweet little girl. Your hopes, your thoughts, your dreams, your heart. Grieving well doesn't mean *detaching* from your dead child. It means *fostering* your attachment to her in the healthiest way possible.

As he wiped his tears, Toby knew what to do.

It was time to paint again.

+++

Jayda met with Pastor Thomas to plan a Bereaved Mother's Day event at the church for the first Sunday in May. They worked on an invite list. Jayda and her mom were on the list and two other moms who were just a little older than Jayda. Pastor knew of some older women with past losses and added them to the list.

"What about Ginny?" Pastor asked.

Ginny was an elderly woman in the church. She had large thick glasses, attached to a shiny chain around her neck. During the winter she wore a long faux fur coat and she drove a car that Toby affectionately called "The Boat". She had been part of the church for longer than anyone could remember. Mostly she was a sweet old lady, although she was passionate about certain things, and could make her voice heard.

"Years ago, when I first started pastoring, Ginny

came by the church office one day. She got talking like she sometimes does. I don't know how we got around to the topic, but she told me something I am not sure a lot of people know. Her first child was stillborn. Full term. A little boy. If I remember right, his cord was wrapped around his neck."

Pastor paused and looked over Jayda's shoulder.

"I'm not sure..." His gaze came back to Jayda across from his desk, sitting in the same seat Ginny sat in years earlier. "I'm not sure I helped her much."

"What do you mean, Pastor?" Jayda was thankful she wasn't with Pastor Thomas and Toby's dad that day in the waiting room. It was clear that Toby had avoided Pastor ever since.

"Well, to be honest, Jayda, I said a lot of the same things to her that I was saying to Toby when..." He cleared his throat, "I told her God had a purpose for all this. I told her that God doesn't give us more than we can handle. I told her that God must have needed another angel in heaven."

"I see," Jayda pursed her lips and leaned forward in her seat. She didn't need to tell Pastor Thomas that those comments could be hurtful. There was a long pause.

"Jayda, I hope Toby can forgive me. Even a pastor can have a lot to learn. And I'm trying. I just don't know what to say." Jayda saw Pastor with tears in his eyes for the first time that day. But it would not be the last.

+++

Not only did every mom on the invite list, including Ginny, show up for Jayda and Toby's Bereaved Mother's Day event, but many of them brought along friends who also had miscarriages, stillbirths, or had lost children in other ways.

Jayda's heart was broken for these moms, but full at the same time, looking over this room *full* of women in the same club, a club none of them wanted to join. Now, she watched her tall, handsome husband at the canvas in front of the classroom at church.

This was Toby's moment. He was in his element when he painted, and he had selected a simple painting of a tree in a field. Each participant had their canvas in front of them. Pastor had approved the funds to make it a free event. The ladies followed Toby's lead as they created their paintings of their trees. Although some of the women protested at first, saying they weren't artistic, now the room was full of talking and laughter. Each mom held a paintbrush.

Toby knew what was next, but he was the only one.

When the tree was nearly finished, he said, "And now, for my favorite part of the painting, and the real reason we are all here. The reason we are all in the same club."

The room grew quiet. Toby stepped in front of his print to obstruct everyone's view of what he was adding to his painting.

When he stepped back, there was a new feature. Dead center on the tree trunk Toby had drawn a heart with an arrow through it. In the middle of the heart was a capital D + A.

Toby stepped aside and faced the room. He laid one hand on top of the other, still holding his paintbrush. He smiled his big Toby smile, and asked, "Does anyone know what that stands for?"

Just before Jayda spoke, Toby saw a thin trail of a single tear streaking down her curved cheek.

"Daddy loves Amani."

There was an audible gasp in the room. Ginny crowed, "Awww, young man. Toby, you got me right here, right in the heart, you did!" Ginny pounded her chest with her small, tight fist.

Each mother added some features to their tree to remember their child. Some were just hearts, some had initials or names, a few had the dates their baby had been born or died or both. Some added birds or butterflies.

Later, Jayda was in full control of the sweet group, and Toby was cleaning up. "I don't think I need to tell you what to do with these prints. None of y'all are gonna put these in a corner. These don't belong in a closet or your basement. You all have done beautiful work today." Anyone else might have sounded bossy, but Jayda's warmth filled their hearts just like it had Toby's when he first laid eyes on her. "You take these home. You tell anyone at home about what you did. You hang this up. You put it someplace you will see it every day. It's okay for us to remember our babies. It's important. And these paintings are one way to remember them."

+++

One week later was Mother's Day.

Jayda had two surprises in store.

When she woke up and went to the kitchen, she found Toby. He was grinning and seemed way too awake. Jayda was headed for the coffeemaker. She had dreaded Mother's Day. She knew she was a mom, but not having any children alive and with her certainly made the day difficult.

The contrast between her grumpy, half-asleep face, and Toby's goofy grin was impossible to ignore.

"What?" Jayda asked.

"Oh, nothing. Happy Mother's Day. I love you." Toby stood and squeezed Jayda tight.

"Okay... What's got you in such a good mood?"

"Oh, you'll see. Are you going to make your coffee?"

"Yes... why are you being so weird?"

"I'm not weird. I'm normal. Totally normal." But Toby couldn't stifle his grin.

Jayda went to the coffeemaker. But her mug was already there, full of piping hot coffee. On the counter right in front of it lay an envelope.

To Mommy, it said on the front.

Jayda gave Toby a sidelong look. He shrugged, acting like he didn't know anything about the envelope. But it was clearly his handwriting.

She opened the envelope, took out a single piece of paper, and sat down with her coffee at their little kitchen table. Toby was sitting next to her, his goofy grin still plastered, and his knee bouncing up and down.

Inside, Jayda read:

Mommy, I am so proud of you. I see what you are doing. I see how you are starting to love all these other loss mommies. Mommies of my friends. There are so many kids like me here. Kids that didn't get to stay. And we all love our mommies so much. I saw the work you did to get all those mommies together last week, and I'm so happy. And all my friends thought it was so neat to see you all together, laughing, crying, and painting. Daddy did a good job too. But I see your heart. I see you loving these other mommies. Mommies like Miss Ginny. Her boy has been here a long time. He's the nicest boy. He loves her painting. He saw his name on her tree. We don't cry sad tears here, but I saw him cry happy tears. Thank you, mommy. I love you. You're doing a great job. Hug daddy for me. He has a surprise for you, too.

Love, Amani

With all the tears in Jayda's eyelashes, she could barely see what her sensitive husband was holding when she looked up from the page.

"What are those?" She reached for a napkin to wipe her eyes.

"Tickets!" Toby announced.

Jayda laughed. She had planned on having a

miserable Mother's Day, but it wasn't working out that way. "Tickets to what?" She tried to have an attitude, but the truth was she loved surprises.

"Airplane tickets. I'm taking my little lady to the beach for a week!" At this point, if Toby could have launched fireworks, he would have. "You know how Ginny lives in a condo on the beach every winter? Well, she owns it all year. Last week, she told me I needed to take you there for a week, and she gave us that week totally for free!"

"Well," Jayda shrugged, "When do we leave?"

Toby's grin grew to full size as he leaned close to Jayda and dropped the final surprise.

"Tomorrow."

+++

Jayda's second surprise came at church. They slid in a little late and sat in their usual spot, between her mom and Toby's parents. She handed cards to her mom and mother-in-law. They handed cards to her, too, each with a sweet smile.

The church was full as Pastor Thomas stood to deliver the Mother's Day sermon. His long robes flowed differently this Sunday. His invocation contained an unexpected confession, followed by a special proclamation.

"This morning, let us thank God for all of the mothers in the room. However, allow me also to ask your forgiveness." The air went out of the sanctuary. *Pastor* was asking their forgiveness?

"There are many of you here this morning who

deserve better from me. I have failed you. But I will fail you no longer." He was using his preacher voice, but he was sincere. The church waited with their breath held.

"Many mothers have children who are no longer here with us in this life. I didn't realize how many of you there are until one special young couple opened my eyes. They have educated their pastor. Little did I know how many pregnancies end in miscarriage or stillbirth. I admit that I have overlooked you in my pastoral ministry. It's not because I was ignorant that you needed care from the church. Quite the contrary, my silence, or sometimes my hurtful words," at this, Pastor Thomas met eyes with Toby's dad, "have come from a place of insecurity that lives within me."

"Last autumn, in a waiting room, a brother admonished me. He helped me to see that sometimes the most pastoral, the most caring thing to do, is just to show up and shut up."

"Amen!" shouted an older woman from the front row, and everyone laughed. Pastor Thomas smiled.

Toby quietly began to cry.

"This week, as I prepared my Mother's Day sermon, I wondered to myself if there were any stories of *bereaved mothers* in the holy book. In fact, I am ashamed to admit, there are many that I have overlooked in the past. Even in the gospel story, I found the story of Zachariah and Elizabeth. The gospel tells us that they were honorable, that they were..." Pastor Thomas's voice was rising and the people were responding, "Yes, the good book says that 'ol Zach and his bride were blameless in the sight of God. And yet,"

Ginny called out, "Tell 'em Pastor."

Pastor Thomas was in full voice now, "This couple," he pointed at Jayda and Toby even though he was talking about a Bible story, "This couple was *blameless*, and yet they were without children. And so, I ask you today. Does God not look with favor on the childless? Does God not look with favor on the grieving heart? Does God's heart not break when children die? Did God not cry true tears when his own son died too young? I tell you, he did. And I tell you, he does. There may not be any magic answers, but if God could declare this couple blameless who had no children, then I too, I too, declare you blameless in our little church who have had to see your child's life come to an untimely end." Pastor, at full volume, made his newfound proclamation, "Despite your loss, your sadness, and your broken hearts, you are worthy... You are blameless. You are loved as a child, just as you love your child."

Toby wanted to be the first one to stand and clap. But he had to settle for being the fourth, right behind his parents and his mother-in-law.

Jayda sat on the pew, no less sad that Amani was gone. However, she was thankful that Amani's impact continued. Amani's death broke many hearts–Jayda's, Toby's, their parents, siblings, and friends. Her death paved a path for Jayda and Toby to help people like Ginny and other moms. But little Amani's power didn't stop there.

Amani helped Pastor Thomas see the light.

+++

Back at home after a well-deserved week at the beach, Toby and Jayda sat on the foot of their bed. This time, Toby waited the full five minutes. Slowly walking out of the bathroom, Jayda could not contain her smile or her tears.

"Looks like Amani is going to be a big sister." She said in Toby's embrace.

During her pregnancy with baby Levi, Jayda started a support group at the church for loss moms. Her mother co-lead the group with her, and women of all ages attended regularly. Pastor Thomas often poked his head in just before the group began. One night he stopped by, gave a few hugs, and asked Jayda if she needed anything.

"I think we're good Pastor, but would you pray for us before you go?"

Pastor sat down at the table next to Ginny. They all joined hands.

There was a long pause.

Then Jayda heard Pastor Thomas sniffle. He cleared his throat. Ginny handed him a tissue and patted his shoulder.

"I think you might have to do the honors for me, Jayda."

Jayda, nearly nine months pregnant with Levi, prayed for the women. She prayed for comfort. She thanked God for all their children, on earth, and in heaven. Finally, she thanked God for giving their church such an understanding and compassionate pastor.

Pastor Thomas left the room with tissues in his hand. When they heard him loudly blowing his nose in the hallway, all the ladies smiled and giggled.

1. Statistics Matter

When we experienced miscarriage, we were both blindsided. Although I knew many people who had experienced miscarriage, it was a new concept for Patrick. There's only one word to describe our initial reaction: *shock*.

What happened next is a common experience. Women and couples who had experienced some kind of loss came out of the woodwork. Suddenly, they were everywhere.

> **When we experienced our miscarriage, we were blindsided and shocked.**

Statistics on miscarriage and stillbirth are a little hard to interpret. That's due in part to the timing of when a woman finds out she is pregnant. That timing will determine when, or if, she notifies a physician's office, and whether or not she will seek medical help if her pregnancy ends unexpectedly. However, a few leading organizations provide insight on how many pregnancies end without a healthy and alive baby that gets to stay in her or his mother's arms.

The American College of Obstetricians and Gynecologists states: "Early pregnancy loss is common, occurring in 10% of all clinically recognized pregnancies. Approximately 80% of all cases of pregnancy loss occur within the first trimester."[1]

A key phrase in this quote is "clinically recognized pregnancies". That means that their "10%" refers only to women who have their pregnancy registered at a physician's office, and also record their loss at that office. This number does not include women who become pregnant and miscarry before they seek prenatal care. It obviously cannot include women who miscarry without even being aware they have conceived. Lastly, the number reflects only *early* pregnancy loss, usually defined as before twenty weeks of gestation. So, stillbirth numbers and infant death are not included.

The March of Dimes, an organization dedicated to reducing the incidence of premature birth, refines the numbers somewhat.

"For women who know they're pregnant, about 10 to 15 in 100 pregnancies (10 to 15 percent) end in miscarriage. Most miscarriages happen in the first trimester before the 12th week of pregnancy. Miscarriage in the second trimester (between 13 and 19 weeks) happens in 1 to 5 in 100 (1 to 5 percent) pregnancies."[2]

So, even before we consider stillbirth or the death of a baby after birth, we know that a significant number of pregnancies will end before a baby arrives healthy into her mother's arms.[3]

The March of Dimes, in the same article, states: "As many as half of all pregnancies may end in miscarriage. We don't know the exact number because a miscarriage may happen before a woman knows she's pregnant."

In conclusion, the rate at which a fertilized egg results in a healthy baby that gets to stay may be 50/50.

Another 1% of pregnancies that survive the first 20 weeks will end in stillbirth, an experience we will discuss in more detail later. These numbers do not include babies who die in the neonatal intensive care unit, die from diseases or chromosomal anomalies, are victims of violence, or whose death is ruled a SUIDS death (Sudden Unexplained Infant Death Syndrome).

Taken together, research indicates that the rate at which a fertilized egg results in a healthy baby that gets to stay may be 50/50.

So, while we were shocked and blindsided when our baby died before 20 weeks, it's a heartbreakingly common experience.

Notes

1. August 29, 2018 ACOG Interim Update
2. https://www.marchofdimes.org/complications/miscarriage.aspx

3. We will often speak only of 'mothers' since the physical experience of the loss belongs to the woman. However, fathers and others close to the baby will not be overlooked.

2. What If My Loss Was Very Early?

A loss is a loss, and a life is a life, no matter how small. We believe the era is over when a woman's grief was minimized because her pregnancy ended early. Your grief should not be downplayed by others.

Your baby's life counts.

Your baby's life matters. No matter how small your baby was when he or she died.

In my (Patrick's) first book, *How to Talk with Sick, Dying, and Grieving People*, I frame life in three phases. Phase One is focused on the future, on hope, and plans. Picture a new high school graduate, with everything ahead of them in life. Phase Two is characterized by struggle and overcoming (this is the phase in which we spend most of our life). Phase Three is when our future has become past, and we will no longer overcome the situation. We are usually in Phase Three only when we are dying or in grief. In Phase Three we focus on finding meaning in our pain (not an explanation, but *meaning*).

When our miscarriage happened, we were *very* young. Not only was our whole life ahead of us, our baby's was ahead of him as well. We were the epitome of Phase One. Then our baby died.

> A loss is a loss, and a life is a life, no matter how small.

We went from Phase One to Phase Three without much opportunity to live in Phase Two. That's the unique pain of sudden death, and every miscarriage or stillbirth is a sudden death. There's no way for a baby to *not* be in Phase One. As parents, we were in Phase One right alongside our little one. When we hit Phase Three, it was disorienting, to say the least.

Maria Teresa Bento Tomas, a researcher on the mental, emotional, and social impact miscarriage has on women, points out several cultural phenomena that help explain why early miscarriage might make more of an impact today than in previous generations.

1. **Earlier awareness of pregnancy** comes via inexpensive and widely accessible pregnancy testing. Women from our mothers' generation learned about their pregnancy when they had a doctor's appointment, a blood draw, and when the lab called them sometime later at home (on a landline). Since the 1980s, women have been able to pick up a pregnancy test on their way home from work on a Thursday and know they are pregnant before dinner. Jayda and Toby were surprised, but elated, when they learned

about their pregnancy *very* early. That made their experience of Amani's death quite different. After all, Toby had mentally painted several scenes, and Jayda was picking out clothes for Amani before they learned that her heart had stopped beating.

2. **There are dozens of apps** available that tell moms, in detail, about their growing baby. This adds to the sense of connection between mom and baby. These apps have become more widely used since 2008. While connection between mother and baby is a positive development, it can add to her sense of loss if the pregnancy suddenly ends in miscarriage.

3. **Pictures for the scrapbook** are now available long before the delivery room. In the time between the birth of our third son and our daughter, 3D/4D ultrasounds became widely available. So, during Kristen's pregnancy with Kelsey, we had an elective 4D ultrasound that provided great pictures of her little face, arms, and legs. Those helped us to be even more attached to her. When a woman or couple has pictures like these before a miscarriage or stillbirth, it can compound the sense of loss.

4. Tomas also argues that **changes in mom's daily habits** create more of a sense of connection between her identity and the pregnancy. In other words, if mom stopped drinking alcohol, started taking vitamins, was sleeping in a

different position, etc., because she was pregnant, it amplifies the effect on her mind when she is suddenly no longer pregnant due to a miscarriage.

5. The bottom line, Tomas argues, is that **bonding might start immediately** for the modern mother, resulting in greater mental, emotional, and social effects if she experiences a miscarriage.

This helps explain why the experience of pregnancy loss seems to have changed from one generation to the next.

Naming Your Baby

Should you name your baby if your miscarriage came early? There is no right answer to this question. We named our baby Stephen Daniel Riecke. We did not know for sure that he was a boy, but we always felt he was. Naming him has helped in memory-making (we have a box filled with special items from his short life, many of them bearing his name, including Christmas ornaments). However, we could have called him "Baby Riecke", or our first baby, and we don't feel there would have been anything wrong with that choice. We have friends who did not name their babies, and others who decided months later to name the baby. There is no indication that either of these choices has affected them negatively. We believe moms and couples should do what feels right to them at the time. For us, it felt right to name our baby Stephen Daniel. Stephen is the name of Patrick's best friend, and Daniel is Kristen's dad's name. Our first son who was born living is Daniel Patrick. We love that his first name is tied not only to his Papaw and Uncle DJ, but also to his brother, Stephen Daniel. This is the name we would have used if he had been born alive. We could have chosen another name for him once he died and reserved that name for a future child. We have friends who did this and are pleased with that decision. Stephen would be an adult now; and while we have never regretted our decision to give him his name, we recognize that's not the right decision for everyone.

Less Frequent Experiences

Some less frequent experiences that occur early in pregnancy have many of the same mental and emotional effects on a woman.

1. **Ectopic pregnancy** occurs when the fertilized egg implants in the mother's Fallopian tube instead of her uterus. There is no room for

growth in that space, so not only will the pregnancy end, but it can pose a serious risk to mom's health.

2. A **molar pregnancy** may or may not include a fertilized egg, but the woman will have an experience much like any other pregnancy. The cells that develop include a noncancerous tumor that usually needs to be removed medically. If there is a fertilized egg, this phenomenon will not allow the pregnancy to continue.

3. A **blighted ovum** occurs when a gestational sac develops without an embryo. Because of this, mom experiences pregnancy much like she would any other time, but there is no developing baby. This situation is usually discovered via an early ultrasound if the mother is receiving prenatal care.

4. A mom who **"gives her baby up" for adoption** experiences a loss as well. Despite the circumstances, she had a baby one minute and did not have a baby the next. Sure, she knows the baby is alive and hopefully better off in some unknown way. And, if you're like us, you usually think of these situations from the perspective of the baby/child being adopted or of the parents who are adopting the child. But what about the mom who is left without her child? This pain can have similarities to the death of a child.

Each of these experiences mirrors the experience of miscarriage. At the health care system where we work, we serve mothers with these diagnoses regularly. Their grief is not much different from any other mother. It can be more complicated. In no way do we think of these as *lesser* experiences of loss or grief.

The point is this. Your loss matters. Your baby matters. Whether a mom miscarries at five weeks pregnant or a mom leans over a hospice bed of her 'baby' when he's sixty-five years old, the loss of *your baby* is very real.

3. A Father's Grief

While our miscarriage was a shock to both of us, Kristen knew many women who had miscarriages or stillborn babies. She attended multiple funerals of infants before we were married.

However, I (Patrick) had no context for this type of grief.

At the time, we were both new college graduates, and we were headed to the mission field. I was an intern at our church, we had good insurance, and we lived across the street from the best hospital in our region (the hospital where I would later lead the chaplaincy department).

You might wonder how all those facts about our lives connect to my experience of losing Stephen. They are connected to me because I felt we didn't *deserve* to have this kind of tragedy. In my mind, we were *good* people who were doing things the *right* way. So, not only did the miscarriage feel sad, to me, it felt *wrong*.

Nearly two decades later, I realize that bad things happen to good people, and the belief that some people deserve grief less than others is not a helpful view. But, at that time, I was angry. I was angry because my son died.

Once, shortly after the miscarriage, I was in our little backyard surrounded by a chain-link fence with our beloved dog, Jackson. I was boiling inside over the sense of injustice. *Why would God let this happen—to us? Why were other people having babies right and left, and the minister and his wife were experiencing such grief?*

It seemed like Jackson was taking too long in the backyard, and when he came close, I kicked him

> I kicked the dog because God was out of reach.

right in the rear end. I had never kicked him before. I loved Jackson with all my heart. So why did I kick him?

I kicked the dog because God was out of reach.

I would have preferred to kick God instead.

(Later, I apologized to Jackson. He was gracious and forgave me.)

So, my primary initial response was anger.

Later, I just needed to talk about it. I even discussed Stephen in a lot of my sermons over the next few months. It's not for everyone, of course, but having a formal way to mention Stephen helped me tremendously. Dads sometimes need an excuse to talk about their baby. We might need a memorial service, or an annual tradition, a grief counselor or support group, to have a "reason" to talk about our grief.

A dear friend of ours, Kavin Ley, has written beautifully about his experience as a grieving father. His book, *Asher, My Son, A Year in the Life of a*

Childless Father, chronicles his grief after Asher was born still. Get his book today if you are a dad in grief.

> **Moms, don't expect dads to feel like you do. We don't. But that doesn't mean we don't feel anything.**

Toby experienced his grief as a simmering rage before his dad put Pastor Thomas in his place. Then he experienced disappointment with Auntie Jean. Later, his grief over Amani was a roadblock, keeping him from painting for several months. Eventually, painting was a pathway for him to express his deep love for Amani.

Toby and Jayda supported each other. Sometimes grief can divide a couple, but that's not necessary. If the couple can allow each other to respond uniquely and take turns being the supportive one, it can bring them closer.

Moms, don't expect dads to feel like you do. We don't. But that doesn't mean we don't feel anything.

4. Faith Matters

We are both Christians. Our faith matters to us a great deal. I (Kristen) decided to go into ministry when I was still in elementary school. In high school, I led Christian activities at my school and church. Going to a college for ministry was an obvious choice for me. My sense was always that Jesus was so good to me, that it felt natural to be a conduit of that goodness to others.

I (Patrick) grew up exposed to faith, but it didn't become important to me until my senior year of high school. Then, a switch flipped. Faith became the most important thing in my life. I felt compelled to give everything to follow God's call.

In twenty years of serving churches, we have seen the collision of faith and grief in many ways. In my (Patrick's) current role, as the director of chaplaincy at Parkview Health, I lead a team of chaplains who respond to traumas, deaths, and fetal demises every day. I avoid the phrase *fetal demise* whenever I can. But, clinically it is an umbrella phrase we use daily to describe miscarriage, stillbirth, and a handful of other situations.

So, imagine, you're a mom who has just lost a baby. You're in an emergency room being prepped for surgery, or you have just delivered a stillborn baby, and a hospital chaplain introduces herself. At that moment, your feelings about faith and your loss might surface powerfully.

When I (Kristen) walk into rooms with our Kindred Hearts program to support moms who are experiencing stillbirth, I don't describe myself as a person of faith. I'm simply a volunteer who has had a loss myself, and I have tools to help mom. However, faith often becomes a point of discussion when I am in the room as well. In the support groups I lead, faith and the varying responses of our religious communities are a common topic of discussion.

All these experiences have provided us with the following reflections:

1. **Many people of faith are lost.** From stories about priests who refused sacraments, to pastors having panic attacks about performing funerals for children[1], one thing is clear. Clergy are seldom prepared adequately to help those in grief over losing a child. This doesn't mean they have bad intentions. They simply lack the tools.

2. **These are watershed moments.** During the experience of loss and the early weeks thereafter, many grieving parents bond with their religious community. Others are filled with anger and feel betrayed by their faith, community, or leaders. Many mothers have said something like "...And that's why we don't go to church there anymore...". Others still

treasure their child's baptismal certificate or pictures of the pastor praying over the family. For those who care about faith and religion, this is often a make or break moment.

3. **The senior leader isn't always the best pastor.** Often the senior pastor, priest, rabbi or imam, did not come to his or her position because of their gifts with those in grief. They might be in that role because they are excellent leaders or public speakers. Those skills don't always translate into these environments. But many congregations have a more experienced woman, or a counselor, or an associate minister who thrives in Phase Three moments. Allow that. It's okay if the primary leader can't serve your needs. Someone else likely can.

Here are some things that congregations can do:

1. **Program support.** Congregations can respond at the moment to the need at hand. They can also plan and program support. Here are a few ideas:

    ◦ Support Groups–Open groups can be joined at any time and function on a regular schedule (maybe monthly). Closed groups run for a defined length, maybe eight weeks, and happen seasonally (maybe every Spring or Fall). Resolve

Through Sharing, GriefShare, and Compassionate Friends are national organizations that help provide resources for local support groups.

- Meal Train[2]–Select a person in your church who will coordinate meals for any grieving family in your congregation. Develop a couple of tips for those delivering the meals. Read Patrick's first book, *How to Talk with Sick, Dying, and Grieving People*, for resources on what to say when you deliver the meals.
- Blue Christmas or All Saints Day–An annual practice of remembering those who have died, young or old, can powerfully weave their presence into the life of the congregation.
- Bereaved Mother's Day Event–We will discuss this option more fully in a later chapter.
- Create a file of sympathy cards. But don't only send them out immediately. Plan to send one on the first anniversary of the miscarriage, knowing that time will also be difficult for the family.

2. **Pay for expenses.** Funerals can be expensive. The parents may have medical bills they did not anticipate. Nothing sucks more than having to pay medical bills and hospital bills but not

having anything to show for it. No one prepares for these kinds of expenses, and they often happen to younger people who may not have many resources.

3. **Check-in on grieving parents.** Don't be afraid to ask how they are doing since the baby died. Use the baby's name. Ask if the holidays have been hard. Ask if they are dreading Mother's Day or Father's Day. Remember that other children don't replace the baby who died. Resist the urge to try to solve the problem of their grief or provide simple answers.

4. **Avoid the five dangerous inclinations, discussed in Patrick's first book[3]:**

   - Defending God
   - Teaching theology
   - Only focusing on the afterlife
   - Cheering people up
   - Praising them for being strong

Pastor Thomas didn't get it at first. He was trying to use tools that are better suited for Phase Two moments. When we are trying to overcome problems in our lives, we want to be encouraged, prayed for, even taught. But when we are in grief, encouragement sounds like mockery, even prayer can be painful, and teaching sounds pious and uncaring.

If you are in grief and frustrated with your faith

community, try to extend grace. They may be completely unprepared and lost. Remember that they are not God. They are only people just like you.

If you are in a congregation trying to help, admit that you don't always know how to do this. Then, approach the grieving with humility and compassionate support. If you do that, you can't go wrong.

Notes

1. Dr. Jon Swanson provides a resource that outlines funerals, including those for children. Giving A Life Meaning: How to Lead Funerals, Memorial Services and Celebrations of Life

2. www.MealTrain.com

3. Chapter 5, "Don't make these 5 mistakes"

5. Logistical Matters

There are a surprising amount of logistical questions that can come up at the time of miscarriage. Over the last few days, Patrick has received nearly a dozen calls from the hospital with logistical, practical questions about miscarriage from chaplains on duty at our hospitals. These chaplains are smart and well prepared. They care deeply about the people they serve. However, sometimes even a trained professional has questions about how things *work* when a pregnancy ends too soon. Perhaps you have needed answers to some of these questions yourself. Or perhaps you will be surprised that some of them are logistical concerns women face when they experience miscarriage.

1. **What if I miscarry at home? Will I see a *baby*?**
    Many women miscarry at home. They start bleeding, it becomes heavier, and their baby, blood, and fetal tissue exit their bodies. Sometimes the cramping is painful, and that may lead them to seek medical attention. Other times, they can remain at home during the miscarriage and check in with their physician later.
    If you miscarry at home, your question may be

what to do with your baby's remains. If you think you are going to miscarry at home and want to avoid the possibility of your baby's body going down the toilet, a commode specimen collector, also called a 'hat', can be purchased at most drug stores. The hat is a simple plastic bowl designed to collect urine when a woman sits on a toilet. It can catch anything that exits the woman's vagina while she is on the toilet. If you are anticipating miscarriage at home, consider using one of these devices (they are very inexpensive) or something similar. Even if you end up flushing the remains, it may give you a chance to examine them first. Depending on how far along you are in your pregnancy, you may or may not see anything that looks like a baby. However, we know women who miscarried at home *very* early and saw their fully-formed baby. Some babies were born still inside the gestational sac. They peeled away that sac and were able to see their tiny baby.

The most common experience may be for the products of conception (baby, blood, and tissue) to end up in a toilet. Sometimes moms don't have much of a choice. If they happen to be traveling and miscarry in a public place, their options are fewer. Many toilets in modern bathrooms are equipped with an automatic flushing mechanism, and it can be nearly impossible to retain those remains before the toilet flushes.

This occurrence can be traumatic or helpful. Some moms may feel that they are glad to simply have *something* to do with their baby remains. Others may be horrified that their baby went down the toilet, purposefully or accidentally.

We simply want to say: this *does* happen. It can be nearly or totally unavoidable. If it hurts, that's normal, and you have every right to feel that way. You didn't do anything wrong; neither did the untold numbers of women who have had the same experience in a public restroom or their bathroom at home. Kristen wants to hug you. Patrick's not much of a hugger.

2. **What are my options for the disposition of my baby's remains?** *Disposition* simply means what you will do with the remains. Will you bury them in a cemetery? Will you use a hospital disposition process? The laws and opportunities vary pretty widely from one place to the next, but here are some nearly universal rights and options for women in this situation.

   ○ **You may choose to have a funeral.** Regardless of gestational age, you have the right to select a funeral home, have a funeral, and burial or cremation for your baby. Deliver what you miscarry (again, whether that looks like a baby or visually looks like tissue and blood), either personally or via a healthcare facility, to the funeral home of your choice. Many funeral homes across the world will perform a very basic funeral service free of charge. In nearly every state and municipality, you have a right to a funeral service. If you cannot afford the services of a funeral home, look for a local organization that might be dedicated to helping fund end-of-life expenses. A good friend of mine (Kristen's) leads a local not-for-profit that does just that for families in our region. Remembering Rowan (RemberingRowan.com) is named after Delaney and Mark's stillborn daughter and provides an inspiring, compassionate resource.

- **You may ask the healthcare facility to make disposition.** If you are under twenty weeks gestation, in most places you can ask a healthcare facility (a hospital or physician's office) to make disposition of your baby's remains. If you wish to know their exact manner of disposition, you have the right to be informed. At our healthcare system, that means burial in a beautiful cemetery in a country setting.

No, the marker does not include your baby's name, but the burial will be respectful and dignified.

- ○ **You may choose cremation.** Cremation can sometimes be a less costly choice, and many parents appreciate this option because they can keep the remains someplace special (an urn, a piece of jewelry, etc.). The more developed the baby, the easier cremation will be. This is simply because there is more to cremate. To learn more about options with the ashes, search "cremation jewelry" online.

- ○ **You deserve to have your baby treated like a person.** Laws are different from state to state and country to country. In our state, the law very clearly requires healthcare facilities, funeral homes, coroners, and others to treat fetal remains of any gestational age just as they would an adult who died. Even if the law varies in your location, you have the right to demand this kind of treatment for your baby.

3. **Can I have genetic testing done?** Yes. Genetic testing can be done on even the smallest amount of fetal tissue. Even if you don't have a fully formed baby in your hands, genetic testing can be performed. A request for

autopsy usually requires that the baby be over a certain size, but genetic testing can be done at any stage. The cost for this kind of testing often falls to the patient. Few insurances cover genetic tests after a miscarriage. Testing seldom explains the miscarriage, but it is an option. Increasingly, the gender of the baby can be determined very early via a blood test for mom.

4. **What is a D & C?** Dilation and curettage (D&C) is a common procedure to remove tissue from inside a woman's uterus. I had a D & C after our miscarriage. I admit that I was both devastated and afraid. It was my first time under anesthesia. No one ever wants to have surgery, but it broke my heart that, much like Jayda, the reason for my surgery was the death of my baby. We chose a D & C because my body wasn't miscarrying naturally (called a "missed miscarriage"). We went home and gave it a little time in hopes that I would start bleeding after the ultrasound revealed that Stephen had died. When I did not, we visited our new physician (we fired our first one because she was far from compassionate—a story for another time). In his office, he told me, "If you were my wife or daughter, I'd recommend surgery." The procedure was pretty simple, and I went home a few hours later. We felt we had done the right thing to prepare my body for any future

pregnancies. If I knew then what I know now, I would have made a different choice. I remember waking up after surgery and asking the nurse if I could see my baby. She told me there wasn't anything to see. I still wish I could have laid my eyes on his tiny body, even for a moment.

I (Patrick) was a nervous wreck while Kristen was in surgery. There were a couple of people in the lobby with me. I don't remember anything they said. I remember wishing they were not there. I'm not an anxious person at all, but I was on the edge of a panic attack as I imagined Kristen not making it out of surgery alive. I catastrophized the scene as I imagined losing our baby and my wife all in the same week. Obviously, she made it out just fine, but my fear was intense.

5. **What about breastfeeding?** If you are far enough along before your baby dies, one of the forgotten occurrences is that your milk may have come in. Ask your doctor or birthing center for information on how to stop the production of milk, or how to find an opportunity to donate your breast milk.

6. **What if I have other questions?** There are local experts everywhere. Unfortunately, your physician may not always be the best resource. Recently, an obstetrician we both respect admitted that he knew how to talk with

patients up to the point of their delivery of a baby who had died. Then he had nothing to offer. That doesn't mean he's a bad doctor; he's the best! But it does mean that his patients who experience loss might need additional help. In our healthcare system, we have experts in unlikely places. First, our chaplains know more about the logistics of miscarriage and stillbirth than any other discipline. That's not normal. Hospital chaplains everywhere are compassionate companions. Not all of them are as knowledgeable as those in Patrick's department. Second, we have a community health worker named Cori who is the most knowledgeable person in our area about pregnancy loss. She used to work as a care tech in our large Family Birthing Center. Her daughter, Norah, was stillborn eight years ago. When she was on the FBC, she was always their first call when there was a loss. Most hospitals have that person. She may be a nurse or doctor, or she may be a tech or a volunteer. Third, Cori and I (Kristen) lead a team of volunteers called Kindred Hearts. More than a dozen volunteers, all of whom have lost a baby themselves, are specially equipped and trained to provide answers to moms in our FBC. We are called in every time a mom is having a stillborn baby. The point is this: wherever you live, there is likely someone who is known as the *go-to* person when there are questions about miscarriage. Ask. You'll find them.

6. Small Connections: Finding Community

Jayda felt more alone than she was used to when Amani died. She was used to enjoying easy connections with other people. But grief can be isolating, and her conversations with her customers, friends, and people from her church became more difficult. She chose to be honest and open about Amani's death. Months later, she even made the purposeful choice at her church to host an event to gather together with women who had similar experiences.

Both of our mothers experienced pregnancy losses. Both of them love children immensely (we each have six siblings!). Both have supportive husbands. But both of them felt like they had to suffer in isolation after their miscarriage. Like many women, they believed the narrative at the time that you just needed to move on and be strong. They did just that.

We could make heroes out of them, and that would be deserved. But we can also accept that the world has changed. Today, there is no reason for a grieving mother to suffer in silence. Here are some ways to connect with other moms in grief.

1. **Support groups–**I (Kristen) help lead two support groups. One is called Healing Hearts and is for anyone grieving the loss of a baby. The second is our Pregnancy After Loss Support group (PALS). Our groups meet monthly at the hospital where Patrick leads his team. A third meets at one of our other hospital campuses. Each group has a large bowl of chocolate, several boxes of tissues, hot drinks, and a binder where we record baby names, dates, and other demographic information. During the holidays we light candles. On Bereaved Mother's Day, we arrange flowers to take home. We paint (like Jayda and Toby), and create ornaments. Some people talk a lot. Others are mostly quiet. We have a private group online to add to the experience beyond the group meetings. Weekly, I find myself on the other end of a table or phone with these parents. They are precious people that have added to my life in so many ways. I love them. Groups like these are worth trying. If you try a group and it's horrible, don't go back, but don't give up until you find a safe place to talk about your baby!

2. **Online Communities–**Find an online community or group near you. There are national groups and many pages dedicated to pregnancy and infant loss. Local groups may be discoverable as well.

3. **Share it and they will come–**We have said many times that if you start to be open about your loss, other loss moms will find you. We don't advocate pandering for pity on social media, but we certainly encourage you to be honest. If you make a post telling the world that you are struggling with your grief, two things will usually happen. First, the person you think ought to care more than others will disappoint you. Maybe it'll be your mom, best friend, or pastor. They will say something that they think is helpful, and it's not. Or they won't say anything at all and their silence will hurt you more than anything they might have said. Second, someone you didn't expect to care at all will provide some meaningful support. That friend that you were never really super close to or a cousin you haven't seen in years will send you a message that might be just what you need. To this day, Kristen and I can list the names of people with whom we were disappointed in those early days. We can also list the names of those people who surprised us with their support.

We said that grief can be isolating. That's not necessary. It can usher you into a community you never would have found otherwise. As we often say, grief is your admission to a club you never wanted to join. Once you join, however, you may find that club to be exactly what you need.

7. Marker Babies

Jayda and Toby knew that Amani would have a marker baby. The woman from their church gave birth when Jayda should have been giving birth to Amani. Now, for the rest of their lives, whenever they cross paths with this child, they will come face to face with a person who is the exact age that their child should be. They will mark the time that has passed since her death by the age of another child. That's what it means to have a marker baby.

We have a marker baby. Of course, our marker baby is a young adult now. Soon this "baby" will graduate from high school, and we will know that if Stephen was still here that he would be moving his tassel from one side to another.

Immediately after my (Kristen's) D & C, I started struggling with sadness when I interacted with the mother of our marker baby. Watching her pregnancy progress was difficult at best. I wanted to be excited for her, and I was. But every one of her experiences served as a reminder of what I had lost.

I (Patrick) did not struggle with any of these thoughts while our marker baby was still in utero. It seems obvious now, but at the time I could not understand Kristen's feelings of sadness and loss when she thought about this other mom and baby. When the baby was born, however, I suddenly understood. Seeing a pregnancy progress wasn't difficult for me, as a man, because I hadn't lost a pregnancy as Kristen had. What I had lost was the opportunity to hold my newborn baby. When I saw our marker baby alive and in the parents' arms, a switch flipped in me. I was angry again. It felt so wrong to me that their baby was fine and healthy, and ours was just... gone.

I have often looked at the marker baby phenomenon as *only* painful. What good could come from thinking about something that someone else has that I lost? In preparation for this chapter, Kristen opened my eyes after nearly two decades.

Having a marker baby isn't all bad.

"Having a marker baby isn't all bad," she said.

"How's that?" I asked.

"It makes Stephen more real to me. It helps me to realize how tall he might be, what he would be doing, and gives me a specific way to think about him and keep his memory alive." She said it like it was obvious. Which, for me, it was not.

I (Kristen) have heard other moms echo the sentiments that having a marker baby in your life can be helpful. It can help us remember our children in concrete ways. Sure, those memories are often bittersweet, but it would be sadder to not think about them at all.

Marker babies are simply a phenomenon to be

aware of. If you realize that another baby, child, or even adult, is a trigger for your grief (or anger), don't deny it. Admit it, at least to yourself. Lean into it. Ride the waves of emotion that the marker baby brings.

8. Bereaved Mother's Day

"When a child loses his parent, they are called an orphan. When a spouse loses her or his partner, they are called a widow or widower. When parents lose their child, there isn't a word to describe them."
President Ronald Reagan

In 1988, President Ronald Reagan declared October as National Pregnancy and Infant Loss Awareness Month. Since then, October 15 has been widely recognized as a day of remembrance for children gone too soon. Beginning in 2010, the first Sunday in May each year has been recognized as International Bereaved Mother's Day. It falls the week before Mother's Day.

Many loss moms feel like Jayda on Mother's Day. She wanted to pretend it didn't exist. She dreaded the day, even though her mother was still living and a special person in her life. Many cultural aspects amplify the pain of bereaved mothers around this time of year. From advertising that includes image after image of women surrounded by living children, to faith communities honoring mothers with living children during their Sunday gathering, bereaved mothers can feel more isolated and excluded on Mother's Day weekend than at any other time of the year. That's why International Bereaved Mother's Day is so important. It provides a scheduled, purposeful way to celebrate moms who have children in their hearts but not in their arms.

Jayda chose to lead an activity on this special day. It didn't erase the sting of Mother's Day, but it allowed her to say Amani's name out loud and to be a part of a community that understood the experience of loss.

Last year, for the first time, I (Kristen) hosted an event for Bereaved Mother's Day. I partnered with a local funeral home and a florist who helped us create our floral arrangements. Some moms simply took them home to display for the weekend. Others shared theirs with their mothers or friends who had also lost children. Please don't picture a room full of crying women. I won't say that we didn't shed some tears that night, but we also laughed, told stories about our lives, and had a great time learning the art of flower arranging. As usual, we stayed much later than planned, enjoying the freedom and safety this kind of setting can provide.

Emmaline's Story

Emmaline never really wanted a family. Until she did.

Emmaline wasn't close to her family of origin, and she never married. That was fine with her.

Emma's career as a nurse practitioner was rewarding and fulfilling. She worked with cancer patients in a doctor's office. The hours were long, and she gave herself fully to her patients and their families. Whenever she felt tired or lonely, she thought of her current favorite patient and rallied the strength to serve these people living with a painful diagnosis.

Life was as meaningful as it was predictable for Emmaline. She enjoyed working with her colleagues, and her patients were grateful for her compassionate and capable approach. When work was extra stressful, she let her mind wander to her next vacation, trips Emmaline often took alone. Her demanding career left little time for friends, and she seldom visited family.

But then there was Bethany. Bethany's warm smile and kind heart always made Emmaline feel connected and cared for. If Emmaline had to pick a best friend, she would have picked Bethany, and Bethany would have picked her. They roomed together a couple of semesters in college, and their friendship was easy and natural. Over the years when Bethany's heart broke over a failed opportunity or friendship, she called Emmaline. Similarly, when Emmaline's studies or work became overwhelming, she called Bethany. While some of her other college friendships had grown distant through the years, Emma's with Bethany had only grown closer.

Bethany and her husband Brad regularly invited Emmaline to visit their small family, and even though they lived hundreds of miles apart, Emmaline visited several times. She was in the lobby when their first daughter was born. Haley was just about the most perfect human being Emmaline had ever seen. Bethany and Brad were so happy, and Emmaline was so happy for them. She couldn't make the trip when Micah was born a few years later, but she met him as soon as possible.

While Bethany was pregnant with her third child, she called Emmaline with a special question.

"Emma, Guess what we just found out?" Bethany prodded on the phone.

"What did you just find out?" Emmaline wondered if they were having twins because Bethany sounded so excited.

"My blood work came back, and we're having a girl!"

"Yay!" Emmaline was happy for her, but Bethany seemed to have more to say.

"And..." Bethany paused. She had a way with

words and seemed to have chosen her next words carefully.

"Yes...?" Asked Emmaline.

"I talked with Brad about this. Your spirit has always kindled a sense of pride inside of me. The way you serve people with cancer is such... such an art. It's a craft. It's like watching an artist at a canvas or a potter at a spinning wheel."

Small tears formed in the corners of Emmaline's eyes. She could feel her face getting flush. She never knew how to respond when Bethany pointed out the obvious impact of her daily work.

"So, I did what all good moms do..." Bethany's tone was playful. "I looked up the name online to see what it means." She didn't say what name she was talking about, but a small lump was forming in Emmaline's throat.

Next came the announcement Bethany had called to make, even though it was still indirect.

"Emmaline means 'industrious'. Or it can just mean 'work'. At first, I thought that was kind of boring. But, *work* can mean something beautiful. *Your* work is something I admire so deeply. And, well, if this little girl inside of me can find meaning in work like you have..." Now it was obvious that Bethany had a lump in her throat, too, as she finally told Emmaline.

"Emma, sorry, Emmaline," Bethany never called her by her full name. "In the hopes that she will also find such meaningful work, would you be so kind as to allow my daughter to share your name?"

"You want to name her Emmaline?" Emmaline was genuinely shocked.

"Emmaline Joy. I'll probably call her Emma, too." Bethany was giddy with joy.

However, Emmaline misunderstood the last two words of Bethany's last sentence–"Emma, too".

"You'll probably call her Emma II? Like Emma, Jr.?" Later she would feel silly for this misunderstanding.

"Well, I like you a lot Emma, but, no, not *Junior*. I mean I will probably call her Emma, *also*." And Bethany laughed so hard she snorted.

The rest of the phone call was filled mostly with tears and laughs and love. When Emmaline hung up, she sat by herself in her car outside of her apartment, imagining what it would be like to meet her little namesake: Emma, Jr.

+++

A few months later, Emma was driving home after working late. Her phone rang again with a call from her best friend.

"Emma, I have something I have to tell you," Bethany said after some small talk. Emmaline could tell her friend's tone was serious.

"First of all, Baby Emma is fine–growing right on schedule, kicking me all the time, and perfectly healthy, as far as we can tell." Emmaline was relieved, but she had a lurking sense that the relief was going to be short-lived. And she was right.

"Me, on the other hand..." Bethany's voice was strong but strained. "Emma, they found something on one of my ovaries. A cyst, or tumor, or something. The doctor called it 'suspicious'. Since my due date is getting so close, they aren't going to do anything more right now. Emma, I'm scared to death. You see things like this at work all the time. What do you think they're going to find?"

Emmaline's oncology training seemed to slip away like sand through her fingers. Her years of experience, which she leaned on so often to help her patients, suddenly felt meaningless. It was just too shocking that her friend might have something serious that she didn't make much sense on the phone that day. When she hung up this time, again in front of her apartment, she could not even remember what she said to her best friend, a friend who was about to face the hardest days of her life.

Later, as the news settled in, Emma knew that it was unlikely that this growth Bethany's physician found was benign. She suspected the worst. She imagined that her warm, wordy, friend with two precious kids and a third on the way–a third that was going to share Emmaline's name–was likely going to be visiting an oncology office very soon that was not unlike the one Emma worked in every day. She tried to block it out, but the picture of Bethany checking into an office, waiting with Brad in a cramped lobby, being called back by a nurse, and sitting on the crinkly white paper of an exam table kept pressing into her imagination. If the news was what they all feared, she wondered how the doctor, or maybe a nurse practitioner like her, would give Bethany the news. Would she get a call on the phone? Would her labs show up online? Or, would her doctor approach the situation with competency and compassion—as Emma always did?

One day, in the hallway of her apartment, when this image and these questions kept pressing into Emma's mind, she squeezed her eyes closed and imagined how she would deliver the news to Bethany.

She could see Bethany walk into an exam room. She saw herself walk in the room with Bethany's chart in her hands. Bethany wasn't on the exam table. She was sitting in one of the chairs, with Brad next to her, her parents were watching the kids. Bethany's shoulders were tense, and her eyes had subtle lines under them.

Emma imagined herself sitting in the small beige rolling chair and pulling up close to her friend.

"I know there's really only one question on your mind," Emmaline said. Then she put her hand on Bethany's hand. Their fingers wrapped around each other. With her other hand, she reached out and took Brad's hand.

In their holy circle of three hearts, three friends, who had known each other for nearly two decades, Emma imagined that she would not even need to say the word, 'cancer', but that they would know because of the tears forming in her eyes as she looked into Bethany's kind heart and darting eyes. Emma imagined herself standing and leaning over Bethany and embracing her, her hair covering Bethany's face and resting on her soft jacket. They would cry together like best friends do when they are sad and afraid.

In her apartment, Emma finally let her heart break. She fell to her knees. She cried. And prayed. But those two actions seemed to be the same thing.

When Bethany called her later to confirm her fears, Emma was more prepared. She was compassionate, but she was also ready to help Bethany get through this. To beat cancer.

+++

Over the next months that turned into nearly three years, Bethany rode the roller coaster that so many people ride when they have a cancer diagnosis. When she was going through her treatments, Emma would order little things online and have them mailed to the house. Sometimes they were gifts to help, and sometimes gifts to make her smile. Once she sent Bethany a pair of socks with cats all over them because Bethany hated cats. Other times she sent gifts of comfort, like a journal tailored to people with cancer, or special hats that one of Emma's co-workers made for their patients.

Often, she included gifts for the kids. One gift she sent to baby Emma became a favorite. The book *Horton Hears a Who* by Dr. Seuss became a fixture in their house for some time. One day, Emmaline received a picture. It was from Bethany. In the picture, Bethany was wearing a blue knitted hat that Emmaline had sent through the mail. Her hair had all fallen out from the cancer treatments. But on her lap sat baby Emma. And in Bethany's hands was this little book. Bethany sent the following note, which made Emmaline laugh:

> The book is great, thank you. However, Emma has really adopted the last line of the book. Now, whenever she isn't getting her way, she reminds us of that last line. "A PERSON'S A PERSON, NO MATTER HOW SMALL!" Apparently, that means we need to be like Horton and listen more carefully to what she wants. Today, she quoted that line in an effort to stay awake as late as Haley and Micah. It didn't work this time, but it has worked at other times.

Emmaline could just picture baby Emma, who was now turning into toddler Emma, stomping her foot, crossing her little arms, and asserting that *a person's a person, no matter how small.*

+++

"I'm cancer-free!" Bethany's voice was tired, but thankful when she called Emma after a much-anticipated test.

Emma celebrated by sending Bethany a gift card

for her favorite coffee shop. The dollar amount on the card was obscenely high. A blessing of being a single woman with a high-paying job was the way she could bless Bethany and her family. Bethany's friendship, however, was a gift to Emmaline that she could never repay.

If there was one thing Emma knew all too well, it was that the description of 'cancer-free' is not always permanent. For Bethany, that description was fitting for less than a year. When the cancer returned, she dove right back into treatments.

During a visit to Brad and Bethany's home, Emma saw the expression on Bethany's face that she had seen on the face of many patients through the years. The expression was one of resignation. Not just determination to 'fight' cancer, if people can even fight such a disease. But a look that simply said, "I'm ready for whatever happens next." Emma had always admired that expression on her patients, but she hated it in Bethany. She tried to distract herself by focusing on Baby Emma, or "Emma, Jr.". She liked to call her "Emma, Jr." because it reminded her of when Bethany called to tell her about her little namesake. It had been a joke between her and Bethany ever since. In reality, Baby Emma was already showing some similarities to Emmaline. She was a bit serious when she was working on something, like a baby puzzle, or lunch. She was compassionate, even toward her big brother. Once, when Micah came in with a skinned knee from the front yard, Baby

Emma climbed up next to him at the kitchen table and patted his leg with her plump toddler hand. Micah would have appreciated it more if she hadn't plopped her hand down right on top of his injured knee.

That same visit, while Emma was pushing Emma, Jr. in the red plastic baby swing in the backyard, she got caught up in her thoughts about her friend's precarity and possible death. She didn't quite cry. She experienced an emotion she could not quite name. It was a mix of fear, grief, and resolve. As she looked at Baby Emma's bright eyes and toddler grin, she knew that she needed to commit herself to her little namesake. She made an unspoken commitment to her prodigy.

"No matter what, you can count on me, Emma."

+++

A few months later, Emmaline made the trip again for Bethany's funeral. She hadn't been to many funerals in her life, so she felt pretty unsure about what to expect. Little did she know how surprising that day really would be, and how it would change her life forever.

Many of the typical things happened. The funeral was at Bethany and Brad's church. The pastor spoke. Bethany's dad wept his way through remarks about a remarkable daughter. There were lots of flowers, hugs, and cards. Bethany was lovely in a simple white dress.

Emma's surprise came before the service had

even begun. A person she did not recognize asked if she was Emma, then handed her an envelope. Her name–"Emma"–was beautifully written on the outside. She recognized the handwriting immediately. It was Bethany's. Stunned, Emmaline looked up to see Haley fall into her dad's arms. They both clutched letters that looked just like hers. Later, another letter from Bethany was read to conclude the funeral service.

Baby Emma sat on Emmaline's lap during the service. She was so thrilled to see "Auntie", as the kids called Emmaline, that Emma was all smiles that day.

Emma could not open her letter until she was back home, in her apartment, feeling more alone than she had in a long time. In the same hallway where she had imagined how she might tell Bethany that she had cancer, the same hallway where she cried/prayed, she finally opened the letter.

In lovely handwritten words, Bethany reaffirmed how much she admired the work that Emma did with people facing cancer, recalled some funny memories, scolded Emma for sending her cat-socks, and reminded her to keep up her good *work* and always look out for Emma, Jr., although she already knew she would.

Near the end of the letter was a paragraph that struck Emmaline right in the heart.

"Sometimes, when you left our house after a visit, I felt a sense of aloneness for you. I don't mean because you aren't married or don't have family close. In fact, I am not sure exactly how to explain it. You're a complete and amazing person without adding anything more to your life. Maybe it's selfish, but I feel like when I die and you're still here, I feel like there will be something missing for you. A void that might need to be filled for you somehow. If I'm wrong, feel free to ignore me. But if you feel it too, maybe I needed to say this."

Emma wasn't sure what it meant, but she did feel it, too. She wasn't mad at Bethany for saying it, because when a dying friend speaks her heart, you can't get mad. But she also wasn't sure what to do about it.

+++

As a medical person, Emma was always curious about new medical advances. When Bethany first faced cancer, Emma researched her particular cancer almost daily, even though she was cautious about bringing up possibilities to Bethany and Brad. The couple of times she did make suggestions based on her medical knowledge, her ideas were thoughtful and well-received.

Many genetic considerations go into the treatment of cancer, and sometimes reading about these topics led Emma from one article to the next, and before she knew it she was reading about something that had nothing to do with her friend or even cancer.

This happened one evening when Emma was home, after having a late dinner by herself.

The article she ended up reading wasn't about cancer at all. It was about embryo adoption.

Here's what she learned: When a family has embryos left over after in vitro fertilization (IVF), they can sometimes be adopted by others. Usually 'left over' means that the IVF process worked for the initial family, they have children now and do not choose to have any additional pregnancies. As a result, many embryos are cryopreserved ('frozen') in labs.

Most articles like this didn't come back to Emma's mind much after she read them. If they did, the information only came back to her when she needed it to care for one of her patients. But, for some reason, the article about embryo adoption stuck with her, even though it didn't impact her patients.

By the time Bethany died, it had been months since Emma read the article about embryo adoption. But when she read her letter from Bethany (a letter she read repeatedly after the funeral), something inside her kept thinking back to that article. One point kept resurfacing, unbidden, in her mind. "Embryo adoption can be a good option for women struggling with infertility, women who have passed menopause, or single women wishing to have a child."

Of course, when she read the simple phrase "single women", she identified with that. But, "wishing to have a child"? Not so much. She never really wanted a family.

"However," she wondered a few weeks after Bethany's funeral, "if I don't want to have a child, why do I keep thinking about this article, and this sentence? More importantly, why was it the first thing that came to my mind when I read Bethany's letter?"

+++

Emmaline knew that Bethany's in-laws lived just a few towns over, so she wasn't surprised when Brad texted to say that he and the kids would be in visiting if she wanted to see Emma, Jr. and the other kids.

Emma turned that opportunity into what she deemed "Camp Emma". Baby Emma spent a long weekend with her. The two Emmas went to the zoo, which they both loved. They also went to the mall, which Emmaline wanted to love, but a crying three-year-old doesn't make for a good shopping buddy. The coffee shop was a hit for both of them, one enjoying a latte, and the other a pastry. When Emma woke up crying in the middle of the night a few times, Emmaline was surprised at how natural it felt to soothe her, and the sense of love and pride she had once she laid her little buddy back down on the guest bed.

All in all, Camp Emma was a success, even though Emmaline went back to work a little more exhausted than usual that Monday morning. Work was long that day, and Emma grabbed dinner on her way home. After eating by herself and taking care of a few chores, Emmaline went into the guest bedroom. There she found a little hair bow that her young weekend roommate had left behind. She picked it up and felt a swell of emotions.

In what felt like a flash, all these things came together. Emma's letter from Bethany, the feeling she had when cradling little Emma in the middle of the night, and the embryo adoption idea that she could not get out of her mind.

"Oh my goodness," Emma said out loud to God, herself, and no one in particular, "I'm a 'single woman wishing to have a child.'"

+++

The process of embryo adoption was easier but longer than Emmaline had imagined. At first, she worried about whether or not she would be accepted, though her fears were unfounded. Once she was in the process to adopt one of these frozen embryos, however, there were a million forms to sign, a home study to be done, applications to complete, approvals to wait on, clinical tests, and confirmations to submit.

Eventually, though, she was... done. After all the phone calls with the agency, she almost didn't know what to do when they told her her application and approvals were all complete and she would be scheduled to have an embryo adopted.

After a few months and about a million doctor

appointments, labs, and shots she was… *pregnant*. She had never thought she would use that adjective to describe herself. But there she was, full of hope, joy, and another person! Sitting at home one night, she pulled out her letter from Bethany. She knew that Bethany was right, and she knew this was the right next step for her. After all, it's harder to feel alone when a little person is growing inside of you.

During Emmaline's pregnancy, she thought about the family who had donated the embryo, her baby. Had they experienced many years of infertility? Miscarriage? Stillbirth? Her heart went out to them, but she felt such excitement at her own newfound family that she quickly forgot how difficult it can be for a child to enter the world safe and healthy.

Unfortunately, thoughts quickly forgotten sometimes return to a person in devastating ways.

+++

"Brad put Emma, Jr. on the phone."

"See her!" Said little Emma. So Brad switched to a video call.

As soon as now-pregnant-Emmaline saw Emma, she could not contain her smile.

"Guess what?" She spoke very plainly so the preschooler would not miss the message.

"What!?" Emma exclaimed.

"Auntie Emma's baby is a little girl!"

Emma yelled something that was mostly unintelligible, but she seemed pleased.

It turned out that Haley was in the room, too, doing her World History homework.

"I knew it! I knew it!" Haley boasted. "I knew you were going to have a girl!" She had always been the intuitive one.

"That's great, Em! I'm super happy for you," Brad said. "I just wish Bethany was here to celebrate, too." He said it so automatically, that it just tumbled out. "I'm sorry, Em, I shouldn't have said that. This is a reason to celebrate, not a time to be sad."

"I think it's probably both, Brad." Emmaline choked back tears. "But now that you made me cry, I'm going to return the favor." Although Emma had a vivid imagination, she didn't have a way with words like Bethany. Still, she gave it her best shot.

"It still feels so wrong that the world is without a person like Bethany. It feels like such a violation. Or like a sin against us all." Brad nodded on the video call.

"I know that nothing can fix that," Emmaline went on, "but there is one thing I want to do." She wiped her cheeks with her left hand as she paced in her back hallway, in front of the guest bedroom she was transforming into a nursery for her daughter.

"I can honor Bethany and keep her name on our lips. And that's what I intend to do. Brad, if you're ok with it, I want to give my daughter her name. I want to name her Bethany."

When Brad had wiped his tears, he told the kids. Micah just said, "Cool," and, of course, Haley already had a sneaking suspicion. Even though she swore she could have guessed that Emmaline was going to name her daughter after her mom, Haley still had tears. A lot of tears.

+++

Pregnancy was not what Emma expected. At times, she felt such warmth and love in her. At other times, she was so tired she slept for eleven hours straight. And she had so many emotions inside of her. She felt like she was starting a whole new adventure for which she did not have a good road map. Little did she know how right she was.

Seeing little Bethany dance on the monitor at her appointments was like watching an episode from someone else's life. Emmaline's co-workers were more than supportive, and she kept working right through the pregnancy. Emma wasn't close with her family, but she dutifully sent updates and pictures of ultrasounds. All the while, she wished she could also share these experiences with her best friend.

Nearly full term, Emma was so tired and uncomfortable, she took off work to prepare for Baby Bethany's much-anticipated arrival. She updated her parents and brother and sent a video message to Haley's phone for all three of Bethany's kids. She wondered what Bethany might say to her, what wonderful words she might offer, having given birth three times herself. But just as Emma's imagination began to fire up, her fatigue took over again, and she fell asleep.

Suddenly, at three o'clock in the morning, Emma woke up with a sense of dread. She could not explain it, but she felt like something was wrong. Like something was wrong with the baby. She reached for the Doppler device on her nightstand and pressed it into the side of her belly. She could not feel the baby move. Usually, Bethany liked to move in the middle of the night more than any other time. That was a big reason for Emmaline's fatigue.

Emmaline got out of bed. In the kitchen, she pulled a bottle of orange juice out of the fridge. She drank it as fast as she could. She started walking up and down the hallway of her apartment. Back in the bedroom, she tried the Doppler again. After 10 seconds, she lost her normally calm composure. She burst into tears. She knew she needed to get to the hospital. She grabbed her coat and keys, forgot her hospital bag, and drove way too fast to the emergency room.

If it's possible to experience life in fast forward and slow motion at the same time, that's what happened to Emma when she hit the hospital doors. Nurses, physicians, an ultrasound tech, and an anesthesiologist flew around Emma. So did surgery staff with all but their eyes covered in light blue scrubs. Soon, she was being put under before entering the operating room.

+++

When Emmaline woke up, her mind was fuzzy.

She blinked several times. Then a nurse with thick, dark red hair and kind eyes came into view.

"Emmaline? My name's Suzi." Emma was trying to ask a question, but she felt like she was underwater and trying to talk.

"Emmaline, do you go by Emma?" Suzi spoke slowly but was not patronizing.

Emma nodded slowly, still trying to wake up.

"And what's your daughter's name?" Suzi asked as she put her hand on Emma's shoulder.

Emma felt her body lurch when Nurse Suzi asked for her daughter's name.

"Her name... Her name is Bethany."

Suzi tilted her head and smiled. "That's the perfect name for her. How did you pick that name?" Suzi was asking questions slowly still, letting Emma wake up gradually.

"My best friend. Her name is... was Bethany." Emma's mind started to focus and panic struck her.

Sensing this, Suzi sat down in a small chair next to Emma. Now they were eye to eye, and Suzi scooted close.

"Emma, is there anyone you would like me to call for you? A friend or family member?" Suzi asked before she gave her the news.

"No. No, there's not. It's just me. What... what happened to my baby?" Emma felt as though she was hanging above a huge canyon, suspended by a tiny thread.

Suzi took Emma's hand.

"Emma," Suzi's eyes were warm, but piercing, and now brimming with tears. "Baby Bethany died tonight."

With those words, Emmaline's tiny thread snapped, her fears were confirmed, and she dropped into that canyon.

+++

For Emmaline, waking up after a c-section and hearing the news that her baby died seemed like a mountain that was impossible to climb. Or, maybe it was a valley too deep to climb out of, or even from which she could see the sun.

After Suzi broke the news, she asked Emmaline a question. While Emma wasn't prepared for the question, she immediately knew her answer.

"Would you like to hold your baby?" Suzi asked in a way that presupposed nothing.

Emma could only nod. Then she checked to make sure she could even move her arms.

Emmaline noticed that Suzi smelled like a sweet coffee drink, like the one Emmaline enjoyed at the coffee shop over the weekend of Camp Emma. She thought it was strange, later, that she could remember how Suzi smelled. But when Suzi leaned over and said, "I'll go get her. She's here in the room with us, in her bassinet," Emma could smell warm memories.

About twenty seconds later, Suzi was back at Emma's shoulder. She was lovingly cradling a bundle, wrapped in hospital baby blankets. A pink hat stuck out the top.

As Suzi looked at the bundle, she had a smile on her face, but tears in her eyes.

She spoke to baby Bethany first. "Here's your momma, sweetie."

Then she turned to Emmaline. "Here's Bethany." And she carefully placed the bundle into Emmaline's waiting arms.

Emmaline first noticed how much she weighed. She was an armful, and sitting on her chest she could feel the body of her daughter press into her own body. Bethany's nose was short and flat. Her eyebrows were thin and fine. Her top lip was like a drawn line, straight across, and her bottom lip was pudgy and wrinkly. Emma didn't notice that she was a little cold.

"She's perfect." Emma heard herself say.

"That's what we all said." This voice came from a young woman wearing scrubs that were a different color than Suzi's.

"That's right. We all agreed, she's as cute as they come." Suzi echoed.

Nurse Suzi had been joined in the room by the doctor, two nursing aides, and a young man who was there to draw Emma's blood after surgery. Their slow pace this morning contrasted sharply with their speed the night before.

There was another person in the room. She was a woman who looked about fifteen years older than

Emma. She was dressed like a professional but didn't have a stethoscope.

After the blood draw was done and the doctor had left, this woman came to the side of Emma's bed–the side where Suzi wasn't standing watch. Before she could introduce herself, Suzi spoke up.

"This is Chaplain Ruth, Emma. She's part of our team. She's going to help take care of you, too."

"I'm so sorry about Bethany's death, Emma," said Chaplain Ruth as she sat down.

"What happened?" Emma finally got the question out to Suzi. She was pretty sure the doctor had explained it when he was in the room, but nothing was making sense.

"Something with the cord." Suzi shook her head, then looked Emma in the eyes. "Bethany had a knot in her cord, and it was caught under her and pressed so much that she lost blood flow for too long. There's nothing you did wrong. It's just something that happened." Suzi could have said more about the clinical information, but she had already heard that Emma was a nurse practitioner, so she stopped there. Besides, Suzi knew all too well that there would never be a satisfying explanation for a baby's death.

"Is there anyone I can call for you?" asked Chaplain Ruth.

Emma's tears came back again. "No. It's just me. And her. We're... alone."

Suzi's head snapped toward the bed. She seemed

a little upset. "You're not alone, baby girl. You've got us. You and Bethany both. We're here. We're here right now. And we're going to be here. Chaplain Ruth is here for you. I'm here for you. And, I shouldn't tell you this," Suzi stepped close again and whispered, "but Dr. Chapman was crying in the hall after he left your room. Besides, in a few hours, another person is going to stop by and see you. You're going to like her. I'll tell you more about her when I come back, but for now, you and Bethany just spend some time together."

The chaplain and nurse left and Emma looked down at her perfect baby. Perfect. But dead. This should not be.

+++

Chaplain Ruth, Suzi, and other compassionate nurses and techs came in and out constantly for the next few hours. Emma learned that Bethany's bassinet was a special one that keeps a baby cool after stillbirth, so they can stay in mom's room for longer.

"We've had moms keep baby for two days after they died, thanks to these little bassinets. Not every mom wants that, but it's good to have some choices," Suzi explained.

Suzi helped Emma bathe Bethany, so she could touch her and see her whole little body. Emma came close to enjoying the bath she gave her daughter. It was the first thing that felt a little normal. She remembered Haley's birth and watching her friend

Bethany as she marveled at all the little baby features. Toes, fingers, ears, hair, nose. After the bath, Suzi brought in several sets of clothes that Emma could pick from to put on Baby Bethany since Emma's hospital bag was still at home.

Eventually, Emma called her parents, her brother, and a couple of her co-workers and gave them the news. It got harder to tell every time. Her mom couldn't come up with anything to say and kept asking Emma what she needed, or what she wanted her to do. That was the first time Emma realized that people don't know what to say when you tell them your baby died. Her mom was trying to be sensitive, but Emma felt disappointed that her mom could not find a way to comfort her when she called. The capable compassion she was getting from the hospital staff stood in contrast to her mother. Her brother just wanted to know why this had happened. He was searching for a better explanation than "tragic circumstance." Her co-workers just kept asking what they could do, how they could help, and what Emma needed.

"I need my baby to not be dead, damn it!" She wanted to scream. If she wasn't so heartbroken, she might have done just that.

Not even two years before this, her friend died way too young and left Emmaline behind. Emma had often talked about how it was *wrong*, or a *violation* that Bethany had died when she still had small children. Those feelings were so strong and real.

They were hot, like anger fueled by a desire for justice. Now, after her stillbirth, the death of her baby on a day when she could have simply been born, healthy and alive, those feelings of being violated by death filled Emma like a fire in her bones.

Emmaline had looked at Brad's name in her phone about a dozen times before noon on the day Bethany was born, on the day she died. However, each time she started to cry before she could dial the number. She pictured those three kids getting this tragic news, and she just couldn't do it, yet. She wished with all her might that she could just call their mom, instead–her best friend. Bethany would know just what to say.

After lunch, a couple of co-workers stopped by for a brief visit and then left. That's when Emma's phone rang with a video call from Brad's phone.

Emma wiped her eyes, took a deep breath, and answered the phone.

When the screen lit up she saw Brad and Bethany's kitchen. In that kitchen, Emma saw not one face, or two, but four.

Brad.

Haley.

Micah.

And Emma, Jr.

It didn't surprise Emma that Haley and Brad had tears.

When she noticed Micah's tears, however, she felt her heart drop again.

Micah just kept wailing, "Not again... Not again..." his forlorn cries shook Emma's soul.

The feeling that this stillborn baby stood in the shadow of Micah's mom's death was similar to what it must feel like to drown under one hundred feet of water.

"Micah, sweetie," Emmaline started. She wanted to say something that would make him feel better. But something different came out.

"It's not right, Micah. No boy your age should have to lose his mom. No mom that young should have to say goodbye to her children. It's not right. It's just not right. And it makes me so," here, Emmaline tried to make herself say that it made her feel sad since that seemed more acceptable. But if there is one thing a young boy with a dead mother deserves, it's honesty.

"It just makes me so angry! I'm so angry that your mom died, and I'm so angry that the baby I named after her died today. Thank you for being angry, Micah. Auntie Emma is angry right along with you."

"Ok," he huffed. "Well, at least we'll be angry together." His mouth curled up on one side. He seemed to appreciate that Auntie Emma was so angry, too. Emma heaved out a laugh before reaching for the tissues.

The part Emmaline was dreading happened next.

Five-year-old Emma stepped to the front of the

camera. Thankfully, Chaplain Ruth entered the room just before Emma came on screen.

"Why, Auntie Emma? Why? What happened to Baby Bethany?" Her words were juvenile, but her soul was experiencing the same shock and sadness as the rest of her family.

Emmaline broke.

She simply came all apart.

She went dark looking into Emma's bulging eyes, searching through the phone for something to hold on to.

Emmaline looked at Chaplain Ruth as if to say, "You've got to tell her, I can't."

"Hi, there! My name is Ruth, and I work here at the hospital where your Auntie is staying today."

"Where is Baby Bethany?"

"Baby Bethany is here in the room with us," Ruth said, plainly, but with compassion.

"See her! I want to see her." Emma made the request that Brad and Haley didn't dare to make.

Ruth looked to Emmaline, who nodded her approval.

A nurse put Bethany back into Emma's arms, but first, the chaplain offered some words to the kids, all gathered around the phone.

"Baby Bethany died in Emma's belly early this morning. Emma did everything she could to get to the hospital so the doctors could help. She's a great mommy. When she got here, doctors and nurses did lots of things to try and help. But Bethany died.

That means she's not breathing, she won't have any wet diapers, and she won't cry or move. But she sure is a cutie. Just wait till you see her little nose." Ruth turned the phone to the bed where Emma was holding Bethany, bathed, and wearing a little yellow and white gingham outfit.

"This is Bethany." Was about all Emma could get out.

From that point on, the kids took over.

"Ohhhhh…. my GOSH!" Micah was the loudest at first. "That's the cutest baby I've ever seen!" He clutched his hands to his chest like his own heart had stopped in joy over the sweet bundle on the screen.

"Can you take her hat off?" Haley inquired.

"Sure," Emmaline let out a laugh.

"Look at her hair!" Haley's big brown eyes were swelling, and her dark eyebrows rose like hot air balloons on her forehead.

The video got blurry when Brad handed his phone to Emma, who demanded a private viewing of this baby. She still had tears on her rosy cheeks when she held the phone out to see the baby.

Emmaline wasn't sure this was a good idea. Her little namesake was only five-years-old, should she be… be looking at a video of a dead baby? There was no decision to be made because Emma had the phone now.

Emmaline held Bethany up and eked out a smile, an act of love for Emma.

Emma's tears seemed to dry instantly.

"She's.... tiny! Look at her tiny hands. She's so cute!" She went on and on, and would not give the phone back to Brad until she had kissed it about a hundred times.

Back on the phone, Haley prayed out loud for Emmaline before they hung up. She insisted. She prayed a lot about the baby, Bethany. But her mom, Bethany, kept coming up in the prayer as well. It made Emma feel like Bethany was right in the room with her.

Chaplain Ruth was praying right along with Haley, and Emmaline couldn't help but feel that those two had a connection at that moment, though they had never met.

After the call, Chaplain Ruth sat silent for a little while before she said, "I thought you said you were all alone."

"Yeah, those kids. They're pretty great."

"I mean Bethany..." Chaplain Ruth tilted her head down and peered up at Emmaline.

"What do you mean?" Emmaline wasn't sure if she meant the baby or her friend.

"I mean that Bethany was clearly a great friend. What do you think she might do or say if she walked through that door right now?" The chaplain nodded toward the door that was Emmaline's portal to the compassion she required today.

Emmaline's eyes locked on the door, and

suddenly, she could imagine her friend Bethany coming through that portal.

The chaplain looked at the door, then at Emmaline. Quietly, she stood, touched Emma's shoulder, then the baby, and said, "I'll leave the three of you alone."

+++

Emmaline imagined her friend rushing through the door, purse over her shoulder, eyes swollen with the trauma of tears, and the rush of a series of interstates.

Bethany's arms fell over Emmaline and the baby, her hair covering Emma's face and resting on the baby's blankets.

She stood there for a long time, leaning over the bed while Emma just cried, with no words necessary. Finally, Bethany stepped sideways and slid her long thin fingers under the baby that bore her name. She squeezed her to her chest.

Kissed her little head.

Sidled her up cheek to cheek.

Dripped tears on her baby blanket.

And finally pulled her back enough to look at her.

"Her face! Her face is so perfect, Emma." She gave Emmaline a little grin, and said, "Must be because she's named after me!"

They both laughed just a little bit.

Then Bethany, ever the one to give the gift of words, sat down, still holding her new favorite baby, and spoke the following blessing.

"This, Emmaline," she said, looking at the baby, "this is your daughter. Your daughter! Your perfect child, loved by you completely and totally. Her death does nothing to change her status in this world. She was knit together by God. She is wanted by you. She is celebrated by me and so many others. Her life, though short, is not without meaning. Her perfect meaning is fulfilled today, in your arms. In my arms.

"Emmaline, you are here on earth. I am here in heaven.

Emma, Jr. is here on earth, Baby Bethany is here in heaven.

Two Bethanies in heaven. Two Emmas on earth."

Emmaline could picture Bethany doing for her baby what she could not do.

She could see her holding baby Bethany, in heaven, both of them totally alive, continuing to love her, cradle her, squeezing her, and kissing her. As the image of her friend started to fade, Bethany leaned over her one more time and whispered to her best friend, "Remember, Emmaline, *a person's a person, no matter how small.*"

+++

That mental image of Bethany holding her baby wasn't the only thing that Emmaline held onto from that first day. The special person who was coming to visit was a woman, a hospital volunteer, who also experienced stillbirth. She had a son, born just short of full term. He had a known condition. So, while the pain of his death was expected for a few months, it was still just as real.

The woman helped Emmaline make molds of Bethany's chubby little hands and feet. They made footprints and handprints and took lots of photos. The volunteer was quite the photographer, and the pictures were so precious. One was posed with Emmaline's stethoscope from work, and a couple of others with her favorite pieces of jewelry.

Finally, the woman gave Emmaline some information on local support groups.

"If you want to try a group, I'll go with you the first time."

Emmaline felt like the woman came close to understanding what she was going through and could see herself attending a group, at least once or twice. The thought of it made her feel less alone.

+++

Emmaline wanted to go back to work the following week, trying to get back to normal as quickly as possible, but her boss urged her to take a little more time. He reminded her that if Bethany hadn't died, she would have taken several weeks of maternity leave. Company policy allowed her the same amount of time, even though she wasn't able to take home a live baby.

The first week, one of her other friends from college came and stayed with her. She didn't do much for Emmaline; there wasn't anything anyone could do. She just sat with her and let her talk.

When Emma didn't want to talk, they went to a restaurant or the movies.

Emma's mom came the second week. And Emma wished she hadn't. She meant well, but she kept saying all the wrong things.

Several times, her mom started sentences with the phrase 'At least'.

Like, At least you had her for nine months.

At least you understand these things since you are a medical person.

At least you didn't have much time to get attached.

At least the baby didn't suffer.

Emmaline hated to admit that she was glad when her mom left.

The third week after Bethany died, Haley came to stay with her for three days.

Maybe it was because Haley was still so young, but her emotions seemed more honest. She cried sometimes when Emmaline was doing just fine. Sometimes Emmaline found herself comforting Haley, but that didn't bother her too much. Other times Haley just seemed edgy and upset.

Haley blurted out at lunch the second day, "I can deal with my mom being dead, now. I've figured that out," Emmaline almost believed her. "But a baby. A BABY. Really, God? Really?" Emma had no words.

Haley read her little leather copy of the Bible a lot. She had a whole set of pens she used to underline and write in the margins. Emmaline felt a little sorry for the poor Bible. It looked like it was once nice and clean. Now it looked like it got hit by a truck–a truck carrying pink, purple, and turquoise ink.

One day, Haley hopped up from the kitchen table with her Bible, looking like she had just learned a secret.

"Look at this, Auntie Emma. You know Jesus raised people from the dead, right?"

"Sure..."

"Well, he didn't raise old people from the dead," Haley announced, as though the implications were obvious.

"Ok..." Emma looked confused.

"He brought a daughter back to life, a little girl. Then Lazarus, who wasn't married yet, and that probably meant he was young back then. And the son of a widow–he reached out his hand to the coffin and raised him to life." Haley's expression looked a little too excited for this serious conversation.

"Ok, Haley," Emma's face was contorted with confusion. "So, what's the point?"

Haley proclaimed her epiphany like she had just won the lottery. "The death of young people pissed off Jesus, too! It made him so mad, he just brought 'em right back to life!"

Slowly, Emmaline started to laugh. Then Haley started laughing, too.

"I know how you feel, Jesus!" Emmaline shouted into the ceiling of her apartment. "I know how you feel!"

Twenty-four hours later, when Haley was about to head home, Emmaline had an epiphany of her own.

"You know what, Haley? I think you'd make a great hospital chaplain–like Chaplain Ruth that I told you about. Do you know what I'm going to do? I'm calling the hospital tomorrow to get in touch with her. I'm going to see if she'll talk with you about how to become a chaplain someday. Your tender heart and thoughtfulness, your prayers, and your intuitive nature–that might just be the perfect combination for that kind of work."

Emma was truly sad when Haley left.

+++

About five weeks after Baby Bethany died loneliness was settling in. Fortunately, about that time Emma attended her first support group meeting.

"If I meet people there that are anything like Nurse Suzi, Chaplain Ruth, and the volunteer who visited me in the hospital, it can't be too bad." She thought to herself.

Good to her word, the volunteer met her at the group that night and introduced her to the group leaders. There were several other women, and a few men, already in the room. They were talking and laughing. Although she didn't expect people to have fun at a grief support group, Emma felt comforted by their smiles.

After introductions, the group began. Emma

wasn't asked to share or forced to answer any uncomfortable questions. She didn't talk at all during her first visit to the support group. Well, not until after the group was over.

The leaders asked Emma to fill out a short intake form for new attendees. As she completed the form, the other participants filtered out and she was left with just the two leaders, who were quietly chatting when Emma stood to return their clipboard with her information.

One of the spaces on the form asked how far along the woman was when her baby died. As Emma looked at the short phrase "full term" she had one of those unexpected moments of intense feeling about the death of her baby–a grief burst.

If the exit had been closer, Emmaline probably would have tried to get out before the grief burst took over. But she made the mistake of looking at each of the leaders in the eyes when she returned the form. At that moment, love for baby Bethany burst forth in a deluge of tears.

It didn't come as a surprise to the group leaders, of course. They had tissues at the ready, a bottle of water, and chocolates (for later). For the next twenty-five minutes, Emmaline told the whole story of her pregnancy, stillbirth, and where Bethany's name came from.

The group leaders mostly just listened, with the following occasional interjections:

"And that's totally normal."

"Oh my goodness."

And

"Which was just what you needed."

Sometimes this last interjection was sarcastic, like when they heard about Emma's mom's comments. Other times it was genuine, like when they heard about Chaplain Ruth explaining the baby's death in concrete terms to little Emma.

When Emmaline mentioned that she had Bethany's body cremated, the leaders could tell there was something deeper Emma needed to discuss.

"Did you have a funeral of any kind?" they asked.

"No. I wasn't sure what to do. I didn't even know I could do anything like that until the hospital let me know I had some options with her body." Emma thought about Bethany's ashes every day.

"Well, what do you want to do?" they asked.

"I don't know, for sure. If I have a service, I'd want my co-workers to come, my friends, Bethany's kids..." She replied. "Do you think Nurse Suzi would mind if I invited her?"

The leaders exchanged glances. They knew Suzi all too well, and said, "She'd probably be a little upset if you didn't."

They offered to support her and help if she decided what to do with Bethany's ashes, gave her some info, and exchanged contact information before Emma went home to her apartment.

+++

It felt good to go back to work, but Emma always looked forward to the support group meeting. In just a few short months she made quite a few new friends and started to keep up with them outside of group meetings. Sometimes it was lunch, or just connecting over the phone or on social media. Some of her new friends experienced lots of early miscarriages and had no living children. Others had blended families with multiple children but had been rocked by the death of a baby. Infertility wasn't uncommon among the group members, and many had spent months or years trying to conceive, sometimes being successful.

This community became like an extended family for Emmaline. She had her co-workers and patients, these loss parents, and the memory of her friend Bethany to fill that void of aloneness.

Several months after baby Bethany died, one of her new friends from the support group presented a small wrapped gift to Emmaline. She explained that although it was a children's book, it had provided her a lot of comfort in her grief. Emma's heart dropped when she unwrapped the book. She recognized the cover immediately. Later, back in her apartment, she wrapped her arms around the little book after reading its concluding words.

A person's a person, no matter how small.

9. Small Wounds: Insensitive Comments

Both Emmaline and Jayda heard hurtful words.

Of course, no one would purposefully wound a grieving person. Many people simply lack the tools to even have a conversation with a person in grief. Words rattle around in the mind and bruise the heart repeatedly, even years later.

Perhaps you have heard some of these comments. Let us react to them with you.

Common hurtful, but usually well-intentioned, comments include:

- **"Everything happens for a reason."** As though there could be a good reason for a baby to die.
- **"God needed another angel in heaven."** Ok, allow us to gather up our collective three degrees in religion and the Bible and say, "That's not where angels come from." We recognize that this image can be helpful to some people if they choose it for themselves. We did not. There may also be a generational aspect to this. A generation above ours seems more comfortable with this image of dead babies becoming angels or even adults who have died. The image of God taking a census of

all the angels, feeling the number is a little low, and then letting some babies die to replenish his supply is seen as problematic by many grieving mothers.

- **"God needed your baby more than you did."** This comment can make God sound sadistically needy and immature.

- **"Move on, it's been (insert number of weeks, months, or years)."** Even today, as we write this chapter, we heard a story of a woman tearfully sharing about a miscarriage that happened *forty years* ago. Which brings us to the next painful comment.

- **"Time heals all wounds."** It doesn't. It can change our grief, but time simply passing doesn't mean anything. It's been nineteen years since our miscarriage. Today, writing this book is one part of our healing. It's an ongoing, never-ending process.

- **"At least…"** At least you got to have your baby for nine months. At least you didn't get too attached. At least you're strong and smart and can get over something like this. At least you have living children. At least you're young and can try again. Any comment that begins with these two words belittles pain that should not be belittled. Kate Bowler, author of *Everything Happens for a Reason: And Other Lies I've Loved,* calls this "brightsiding". As a person living with stage four cancer, she abhors when people tell her to look on the bright side, or start statements with "at least". Emmaline's mom thought she was trying to cheer her daughter up. Because sad people need to be cheered up, right? Wrong. It's okay to be sad.

- **"Trust God."** Let's be honest, grief is the ultimate trust-teacher. Ed Dobson, a long time pastor, as he was nearing the end of his life due to crippling ALS, gave one last sermon. People kept telling him to trust God. In speech so garbled it was almost impossible to understand, he said, "I want to ask them. What do you think I am trying to do?"

- **"If there is anything I can do, just let me know."** Oh great, it's not only my responsibility to carry the heavy weight of grieving my child, now I have to tell you how to help me. An alternative is to say "I want to bring you dinner. Do you have any dietary restrictions I should be aware of?" Or, "I'm going to call you next week to talk about how you are doing. If you don't feel like talking, just don't answer. If you do, I'll make sure I have plenty of time."

We are sorry to say that this is *the* most common experience of those grieving the death of a baby. Although their experiences of loss vary widely from one to the next, their experience with other people always includes thoughtless comments like these.

The acknowledgment that no one means to be hurtful does little to lessen the pain.

If you are grieving and struggling with one of these comments someone has made to you, we are profoundly sorry that happened. It's okay to be angry and hurt. Please don't let these comments dominate your thoughts or emotions. Be aware that they hurt you, and decide you will not let them define you or your grief. If an insensitive comment is still causing you angst, share your feelings with a trusted friend, lay your burden down before God in prayer, or find a capable counselor who will help you process the pain.

10. Honest Emotions

Emmaline benefited so much from Bethany's family and their honesty. They learned from Bethany's sickness and death to feel their emotions openly as they came.

Brad was honest with Emmaline when he said that he wished Bethany was still there.

Haley was honest with her when she expressed how upset she was at God for allowing a baby to die. She was honest when she doted over baby Bethany on the video call. She was also honest when she exclaimed that "Dead young people piss off Jesus, too!" in Emmaline's apartment when she came to visit.

Micah letting out his loud cries when the baby died broke Emmaline's heart, but it also gave her permission to feel what she was feeling. She was angry. She was angry that her best friend died and that her baby died. She had a deep sense of "That's not right!" that needed to come out in words.

Finally, five-year-old Emma was sad, mad, and happy all in the same video call. The younger we are, the more honest we are

When we are sad, we need to ride the waves of our emotions.

about our emotions. Age and "maturity" teach us to

mask our real feelings. While that might be helpful when we are at work or the grocery store (we might prefer to avoid being weepy at certain times), if we can't let out our true, raw emotions from time to time, they will eat away at our insides.

Emmaline's imagination was a friend to her. First, she imagined giving her friend Bethany the news that she had cancer. That helped her be more prepared to support her later on. Second, she could imagine her deceased friend coming in and loving her and her stillborn baby. That imagination wasn't something to avoid, it was a gateway to her honest emotions.

When we are sad, we need to ride the waves of our emotions.

Grief bursts are unexpected moments when grief suddenly overwhelms you.

In the Bible, the book of Psalms is very honest. In some places, the writer asks God to tear his enemies limb from limb. In other passages, he describes his bed as "soaked with tears". Reading Psalms or the book of Lamentations (also in the Bible) out loud can be an effective way to connect with your honest emotions. Mark Vroegop has written a book on this very topic after the stillbirth of his daughter. It's entitled *Dark Clouds, Deep Mercy*, and leads the reader through Psalms and Lamentations.

At her first support group, Emmaline experienced

a grief burst. Grief bursts are unexpected moments when grief suddenly overwhelms you and you "break down". Just that phrase, "break down", tells us something about how we view grief. A grief burst is natural and can be triggered by a thought, memory, question, smell, taste, or a song.

Remember, though, that honest emotions won't all be sad. One of my (Patrick's) favorite experiences, when I speak on grief, comes at the breaks or the end of an event. That's when people come up and tell me about people they have lost in their lives. It might be a story about a dad or spouse or grandchild who died. Inevitably they talk about not only their death but also their life and their memories. While these memories are limited when it comes to babies, it's normal for our emotions to include happy feelings in addition to sadness. I can't tell you how many times, while people are telling me stories, their tears and laughter mix together.

Experiencing honest emotions, including grief bursts, doesn't mean you are weak or "having a hard time coping". It means that you love the person you lost. On the other hand, you will likely experience a full range of emotions, not just sadness. And you're just being honest about how you feel at that moment.

So, don't let other people tell you how you *should* be feeling. Just ride those waves of whatever you feel today.

11. Support Groups

Groups are not for everyone, but support is needed by all. So if your community offers infant loss support groups or other grief support groups, this may be a helpful resource for you. When Stephen died, we lived in a large city. At the time I (Kristen) worked at the large library system, so I spent my break times looking desperately for books on the subject. I found a book or two in the "self-help" section with very little information on the subject of infant loss. I was desperate to find people who "got it". My faith community was outstanding. Women came out of the woodwork to offer their support and personal stories of loss. As time went on, the lives of other people moved on, and I felt left behind, still carrying the heaviness of my grief.

The summer after Stephen died, we relocated to a small town in southern Indiana. It was there

> **Groups are not for everyone, but support is needed by all.**

that we found ourselves in a cozy conference room on the first floor of that small-town hospital talking about our dead son. We only attended that pregnancy loss support group for a few months. However, those sweet times were like a shot of hope into my depleted system. Fast forward a dozen years, and I found myself with an invitation to help revamp and co-lead the infant loss support group at the health system where Patrick now works. When I met Cori McKenzie, a coworker who also volunteered to serve this group, we became instant friends–kindred hearts. We renamed the group *Healing Hearts Infant Loss Support Group*. Our first meeting was small, just a few attendees. But, that first group launched us into over five years of monthly meetings that have grown to include a Healing Hearts group at another hospital campus, a PALS (pregnancy after loss) support group, and most recently gave birth to a program that I help coordinate called Kindred Hearts.

Each meeting begins with the following instructions:

> *Please introduce yourself, and tell us what brought you here tonight. Feel free to share as little or as much as you would like. Please know that this as a safe place to talk about your baby.*

As leaders, we have worked hard to provide a nonjudgmental space where people can share without fear of shame or condemnation. We have chocolate and tissues at every meeting. Some months just a few attend, and that allows more intimate conversations. Other months, we add extra chairs to accommodate everyone. We've met parents whose babies died last week and parents whose babies died years ago. They come alone, with their spouses or significant others. They come with grandmas, aunts, coworkers, friends. They come at the prodding of their physician, midwife, nurse, therapist, pastor, or another member of this club no one ever wants to join! To this day we have over sixty members on our private Facebook page and many more who have attended some of our special events. We provide free resources, books, publications, online forum suggestions that others have found helpful. We gather annually for a Christmas candle-lighting service, a Bereaved Mother's Day event, and a Walk to Remember each October during Pregnancy and Infant Loss Awareness Month. Sometimes, we just get together for the fun of it! Friendships have developed, joys and sorrows have been shared. Tears are usually shed, but laughter also echoes through our meetings.

> **I know, personally, the courage it takes to attend a support group.**

I know, personally, the courage it takes to attend a support group. Some attendees only make it as far as the parking lot for several months before they finally come inside. We have had many people admit that they didn't want to come at all but are so glad they did. We get it! We ALL get it! That's the power of a group like this. Although each of our stories is unique and the pain and struggle surrounding the death of each baby is different we also share a bond that cannot be changed-our babies died, and we now need to learn how to parent them from this side of heaven. It's a lonely journey, if not for the support of others.

Stephen would have been 19 years old this April, so I am easily the oldest member of our support group. Therefore, I have the privilege of standing on the other side of the deep, dark valley of death that group members find themselves in. I see myself waving my arms and shouting to them, "You can do it! You will find your way, you will survive! Look at me! I made it, and you can too!" That is the power of support groups, sharing our journey as we navigate, survive, and thrive in this strange, unwelcome land we now live in, life after a baby dies.

12. Memory-Making in the Hospital

In the shock and fear of what is happening, some parents don't choose to see or hold their baby. They just want the nightmare to end as quickly as possible. However, it is in those critical moments that we need to slow down and soak in what limited time we may have with our children. The fear of what our babies will look like is often unfounded. I (Kristen) have seen pictures of a friend's baby delivered at home at 8 weeks gestation. Mom carefully tore open the sac and spent time with her daughter. She was beautiful! All her parts were there, just in miniature form. No matter how small, this is your baby, your hopes, dreams, and future. This is the only time you get to make memories that must last a lifetime. While these might not be for everyone, here are some ideas about making memories with your baby.

Taking pictures

I encourage parents to take as many pictures as possible. Our hospital has a quality camera that was donated by Gwen's mom, Sarah. She only has a few low-quality pictures from mobile phones. She wanted to make sure future, grieving families had better. There is also a national organization called Now I Lay Me Down To Sleep[1], whose photographers are specially trained to take stillborn photos. They professionally edit the photos, and their services usually come free of charge.

When I help take pictures, I always ask parents if there is a piece of jewelry or a special item I can photograph with the baby. There will only be a few tangible things your baby will have touched. So, taking pictures with these special items can be therapeutic. Emmaline's photos of Bethany, posed with her stethoscope, held meaning for years to come. When she returned to work, she maintained a sense of connection to Bethany by carrying the stethoscope around her neck.

Are there items that hold significance for you, like a stuffed animal for reference to size, a family heirloom connecting the generations, or another special gift? All of these things can be forever memorialized in photographs with your baby.

Reading a book

Our friend, Tim, couldn't wait to read *The Hobbit*, by J.R.R. Tolkien, to his daughters when they got older.

Knowing he wouldn't be able to do so with Norah, he took the time to read a chapter to his daughter in the hospital. Other family members can read to the baby as well. Maybe Grandma has a special book she reads to all her grandbabies. Do your living children have a favorite bedtime story you could share with this new baby, connecting them all to the same book? Doing a normal thing like rocking and reading to your baby is an opportunity to create a lasting bond.

Listening to music/watching a show

Did you play music to your unborn baby? Were you looking forward to sharing your favorite band, worship song, or lullaby? Music connects like nothing else. So, pull up your playlist, and enjoy a special moment of music together. Maybe every week you snuggled on the couch for your favorite show or looked forward to introducing your tiny fan to your favorite sports team. Pull up an episode or previously played game and make that memory. Now, every time you do this in the future you can connect it to this moment in time.

Dancing together

Dads often look forward to the day they will attend a daddy-daughter dance or even dancing with their daughter on her wedding day. Take a moment to dance with your precious child. Choose a special song for just the two of you, or dance with her to the song you and her mamma shared on your wedding day.

Bathing/Dressing baby

These normalizing activities can be done in the room. Parents or other family members can help, too. Using baby wash you can gently clean baby and even wash their hair. If the baby is tiny, you can gently rinse him or her in a sink or a small basin. The changes in your baby's skin and appearance can be upsetting. Ask your care team for guidance. You can decide to put on a regular diaper or a cloth diaper. The organization Teeny Tears[2] can provide healthcare facilities with tiny flannel diapers and matching mini-blankets. Teeny Tears provides two diapers with each set; one for baby to wear, and a duplicate for families to take home. Depending on how long ago the baby's heart stopped beating, his or her skin could be sticky, or even begin peeling.

We want to be as gentle as possible with their delicate skin. If necessary you can use gauze and other means of wrapping the baby's abdomen before dressing him/her.

Swaddling

There are very few items that will physically touch our children on this side of heaven. If you choose to swaddle your baby in a blanket or wrap, that item may bring comfort to you in the future. Any item that baby uses will eventually need to be washed, due to the birth fluids that will transfer to the fabric. Keeping this in mind, you may want to use the hospital blanket as a first layer, next to the baby's skin. For extremely lightweight babies, an extra folded hospital blanket or burp cloth can be placed behind the baby's back for support before swaddling.

Footprints (gifts)

Getting footprints is a sweet and relatively simple way to provide memories. You can use ink and put footprints in a variety of places. You can put them in the baby book, on several pieces of cardstock, on a decorative birth certificate or card provided by the hospital. You can also use inkless pads or regular ink pads. Footprints provide an accurate size of your baby's feet and sometimes hands too. Oftentimes parents use these exact prints to get a tattoo in memory of their baby or have jewelry made with a replica of the prints. We have taken prints of baby's feet and made special cards to personalize gifts for siblings, grandparents, or other loved ones left behind. Of course, the larger the baby's feet, the easier these gifts are to create. It can be difficult, or even impossible, to get good prints for babies under sixteen weeks gestation.

Imprints

Impressions of baby's hands and feet can be made with simple air-dry clay. Crayola Model Magic works well for these projects. When Kindred Hearts volunteers serve a mom, we roll the clay into a ball and flatten it to create a circle. Leaving ink on the baby's feet when making an impression in the clay can accentuate all the tiny details.[3]

Plaster molds

Plaster molds can be made to recreate 3D versions of the baby's hands or feet. The plaster molds take time to dry before families can take them home, can be tricky to use, and are certainly fragile. However, a replica of your precious baby's hands or feet can provide connection, unlike simple footprints or impressions. Again, creating molds for a baby under twenty weeks gestation can be a challenge. Many funeral homes also provide this service before cremation or burial.

3D models

We also have a new opportunity to create an exact digital replica of the baby's feet or hands through 3D printing. We use a very expensive scanner, but the files can be saved for future use, and multiple copies can be created.

There are many ways to make memories with your baby in the limited time you have, whether at a hospital or home. Nothing will take the place of your child. But making memories in concrete ways will foster your connection with them in the years ahead.

Notes

1. nowilaymedowntosleep.org
2. teenytears.org
3. Crayola modeling material in small individual packages work well

13. Compounding Grief

Emmaline was still grieving the death of her best friend when she became pregnant with her daughter. When her baby was stillborn, the feelings of the loss of her friend came back to the surface.

Why do we grieve? We grieve because we have lost something. In his book, *Life After Loss*, author Bob Deits tells a story from his life as a pastor. On the same day, he learned of two very different losses. First, several men working in a mine nearby were killed when their mine caved in. While Deits was certainly sad to hear the news, he did not know any of the men personally. Later that day, Deits' cat died. When he learned about his cat, he cried. He had not cried about the miners. His first reaction to his own emotion was that something must be wrong with him. Why, especially as a pastor, could he cry over a pet but not over the men who left behind spouses and children?

As Deits realized, a person can cry over a cat and not over a nearby tragedy because we grieve when we lose something. Since he didn't know the miners, he had not personally lost anything. That doesn't mean we don't care when we hear these stories. We can empathize and be sad, even devastated. But the experience of grief is reserved for times of personal loss.

Emmaline had lost a great deal when Bethany died. She lost a great friend, someone who made her feel safe in the world. Her connection to Bethany's kids changed once she was gone. And, she lost all the wonderful words that Bethany could speak to her.

When Emmaline experienced a second profound loss, her grief over the loss of her friend suddenly intensified, as though she was experiencing the loss all over again. She wished she could have Bethany come rushing through that door and fill the void that was created when she died.

Emmaline's two major losses came fairly close together. We might be tempted to think that grief would have accumulated less if they had been decades apart. Many theories of grief point to going through stages, or processing grief. Those theories, while they acknowledge that there is no time frame for grief, leave us with a sense that the passing of time is nonetheless a key element in avoiding compounding grief, or cumulative grief.

We disagree with the theory that "time heals all wounds".

Grief and loss exist with only a partial relation to time.

That's why people like Jayda's mom can get caught up thinking about a loss from thirty or forty years ago when a new loss presents itself.

All your grief is connected, just beneath the surface. If your previous loss was recent, they are connected. If your previous loss was a lifetime ago, they are connected. Here's the real surprise. It's ok. It's sad, and it feels wrong, but what did Emmaline experience? With her gifted imagination, she experienced a connection between her baby and her best friend. A connection they would never have experienced if baby Bethany hadn't been stillborn.

This is a complicated topic, on which not much work has been done. But here are our conclusions from being a part of the grief journey of thousands of people and families.

1. All your grief is connected.
2. New grief will likely make you think about previous losses in a new way.
3. At times, you may feel sadder about the previous loss even while you are in the throes of grief over the new loss.
4. The death of a baby through miscarriage or stillbirth can reopen a wound from losing your mom, dad, or anyone close to you.
5. Miscarriage or stillbirth can connect you again to the death of your brother or sister.
6. The degree to which all this connection occurs is beyond your control. Do not attempt to avoid it or conjure it if it's missing.
7. The connection is not to be feared.

Grieving a previous loss anew when a more recent loss occurs is a way you can honor both people. If your mom died before your baby, it's only right that you are thinking about your mom while you grieve your pregnancy loss or stillbirth. Wouldn't you be a little disappointed if you didn't?

Infertility and repeated pregnancy loss

We purposefully aren't directly covering infertility in this book, because it's a huge topic. We experienced a very brief time when we sought the help of doctors for infertility. It gave us just enough of a taste to know how fraught the experience is. For the woman who can never get pregnant, there is the constant tension of wanting and not getting. For the woman who gets pregnant, but regularly loses the baby, there is the pain of having but not keeping. With each pattern (either of infertility or loss), the tension can grow. We add this brief note on the topic under the heading of compounding grief for obvious reasons. But since it wasn't our experience, and we only periodically serve women in this situation, we have chosen to let other voices with greater knowledge speak.[1]

That feeling you have when losses compound, one after another, can be overwhelming. Avoiding your feelings won't help. Your losses and your grief are all connected. While communities and sources of support for infertility and those for miscarriage and stillbirth overlap, they are not identical. If you are experiencing infertility, help is out there. Your needs and feelings are real and significant.

Notes

1. A good resource on this topic for people of color is Fertility in Colour

14. Funeral for a Stillborn Baby

We've both been in the chapel of the largest hospital in our health system many times. One visit sticks out in both of our memories. On that afternoon, a tiny casket sat at the front with the lid open. A baby who was born too early had died. Through a very unusual set of circumstances, the baby's funeral was held at our hospital. As staff gathered around for his funeral service, a few things became obvious to us.

1. **Funerals for babies are hard.** Just the image of a tiny casket is unsettling. As Emmaline said, it just feels *wrong*. Many of us are uncomfortable at funerals for adults, let alone a funeral for a little one like this.

2. **Babies are sweet.** You know that feeling everyone has when they see a baby in the grocery store or at church? We are drawn to babies because they are cute, innocent, and sweet. That doesn't suddenly go away when they die. Sure, they may be harder to look at in some ways because their bodies tend to break down a bit more than adults. However, as our friend Cori McKenzie says, they always look like a baby. As a society, we love babies. Going

to a funeral for a baby has that similar characteristic.

3. **Children will surprise you at funerals.** When our children have gone to funerals or visitations for babies, they are so much more comfortable than the adults in the room. We often remember that the first funeral for a baby that we attended with our kids was a beautiful experience. They went right up to the open casket, without recoiling whatsoever. They doted on the little boy, talking about how adorable he was.

4. **Baby funerals are different.** The chaplains I (Patrick) work with serve patients at the end of their life every single day. The team I lead responds to a death at our large health system on average every six hours, around the clock, 365 days a year. At this point, we are pretty comfortable around people who are dying or have just died. That being said, all our chaplains know that babies (and all children) are just different. It's out of the natural order. Baby funerals are much the same. Even for people who are more comfortable at funerals, funerals for children affect us all differently. That's okay. They should.

5. **Ministers may not know what to do.** Aren't we thankful that pastors and clergy don't have to perform funerals for children or babies very often? Of course. However, that also means

that they lack the tools to do this well. I (Patrick) recommend a book by my colleague and friend, Dr. Jon Swanson to help prepare for a funeral of any kind, including a funeral for a baby. His book, *Giving a Life Meaning*, helps the reader prepare to lead a funeral. Jon and his wife Nancy buried their daughter, Kathryn, when she was five weeks old. So while Jon has lots of professional practice, he also knows some of these feelings firsthand.

6. **Consider a graveside service.** If you are burying your baby, having a short graveside service can be powerful. First, it clearly shows every person who attends the location where your baby will be buried. Later, you might find that someone stops by to remember your baby who might not have if they didn't already know the location. Second, it gives a special quiet moment together as a group before the "formal" grieving is over for the day. Being at the graveside can affect our emotions differently than sitting in a funeral home or place of worship. Third, the kinetic energy of standing, walking, processing with a motorcade, and walking to a graveside where you stand together in grief is indescribable, yet significant.

7. **Consider a funeral dinner.** During the formal memorial service, funeral, graveside service, or whatever you choose, there is usually a sense

that only one emotion is appropriate–quiet sadness. If you choose to have a funeral dinner afterward, it can allow the range of emotion to increase. Laughter can feel appropriate, talking gets louder, stories might be shared, plans made, etc. It allows the parents of the baby and every attendee to incorporate the death and life into everyday life. A dinner feels more "normal" than a funeral. We know how to eat well. We don't always know how to grieve well. So, allowing eating in addition to a funeral can be helpful to everyone.

There's no right or wrong when considering a funeral, memorial service, celebration of life, graveside service, or funeral dinner after a baby has died. The right thing to do is what will help you long term. However, at that point of grief and loss, it can be hard to effectively assess your own needs. Trust those who care about you to help you decide what to do.

Timing is always a question. Since the death of a baby is seldom anticipated for very long, deciphering the next steps can be disorienting. Like Emmaline, you might not know what options even exist until the trauma of loss is already upon you. Her workplace was understanding and supportive. Not all are so generous. Especially after an early miscarriage, some employers might expect you to come right back to work. Ask about company policies so you can know your rights. If you choose cremation for your baby the timing of a service can be more flexible. Emmaline can still choose to have a service even months after baby Bethany's death.

15. Finding Meaning

In my (Patrick's) second book, *How to Find Meaning in Your Life Before it Ends*, I examine ways to find meaning during life's most difficult moments. Emmaline was certainly in the most difficult moment of her life the morning that baby Bethany died. She was grasping for meaning, not an explanation, but a feeling like baby Bethany's life still mattered.

> **"Formally or informally, finding a way to express some important words can be a pathway to finding meaning in suffering."** *–How to Find Meaning in Your Life Before it Ends,* **Patrick Riecke**

One way Emmaline found meaning was through imagining what her best friend might have said to her if she had not died. She could hear her saying, "Two Emma's on earth, two Bethany's in heaven." Bethany found her meaning by expressing words when she wrote letters to her friends and family before she died. Her letter to Emmaline changed her life. Do you recall when Toby found a way to use Amani's voice to speak words to Jayda that she needed to hear? Words have a powerful effect.

The second major way to find meaning is by

giving gifts. Receiving a special gift can make a major impact. My mother gave us a baby bootie that she made into a Christmas ornament to honor Stephen. That's still a special gift that we take time to recognize each Christmas. When her friend Bethany was sick, Emmaline sent lots of gifts that held meaning. And when her new friend from the support group gave Emmaline that special children's book, she could feel the weight of how meaningful it was.

The third and final category of ways to find meaning is actions. Doing certain things can connect us with meaning. In the case of a stillborn baby, most of these actions will be memory-making activities like pictures, molds, footprints, holding the baby, etc., that Kristen has already spoken of so well. My previous book contains a long list of similar activities that help us find meaning as we grieve.

16. Small People Doesn't Mean Small Grief

I think my (Patrick's) favorite person in Emmaline's story is Micah, Bethany's adolescent son. He does two things I love. First, he laments. Mournful cries like his when he learned that baby Bethany had died just three years after his mother's death shake the soul. *Forlorn* is a seldom-used word that appropriately describes his response. He cries out with honest emotion, "Not again, not again!"

Then, when Emmaline shares his anger, he replies with a huff and a smile, "Well, at least we will be angry together." Later, when the kids see baby Bethany, Micah is the first and the loudest, "Oh my gosh! That's the cutest baby I have ever seen!" He's honest. He's raw. His grief isn't smaller than anyone else's just because he's a kid. And it isn't muted because he's a boy.

We have three sons. Because of our work, they are more aware than most when it comes to miscarriage and stillbirth. When their favorite aunt (sorry to the others) experienced miscarriage twice in a short period, our three teenage sons reached out to her directly. They told her themselves how excited they were for her to have a baby, and then how sad they were when those pregnancies ended. We didn't tell them to text their Aunt Mimi or what to say when we saw her next. They felt sad, and a little angry, so they told her.

My (Kristen's) favorite character is Haley. As a teenager, I was a lot like Haley. Unfortunately, two of my church leaders[1] had stillborn babies and one of my cousins, Kyle, died as a toddler. Therefore, I attended three funerals for infants before I even graduated from high school. I was comfortable being with them in their grief and letting mine be seen as well. I prayed hard for them with my youthful soul and found comfort for myself and them in the word of God. I'm thankful that those youth group leaders who experienced stillbirth allowed me to learn from their lives and grief. Like Emmaline's revelation that Haley would make a great chaplain, these leaders, in their grief, helped me to see a part of how God created me. He created me to join with others in grief and to shoulder that grief alongside them.

However, many will say that their favorite little person in this story is little Emma, or "Emma, Jr.". Her stubborn and loving ways are endearing. Her joy at sitting with Auntie Emma during her own mother's funeral and later insisting on seeing baby Bethany and "kissing" her, give us insight into the response of children to death and loss.

Chaplain Ruth was forthright with the children

before they saw the baby. First, she told them baby Bethany had "died". She didn't say she fell asleep or that she had passed. Children, especially young children, need to hear painful news in concrete terms. Using euphemisms is confusing at best and terrifying at worst. We have heard stories of children who were

> **Children, especially young children, need to hear painful news in concrete terms.**

afraid to go to sleep for months after being told that a dead person was "sleeping".

Second, Chaplain Ruth described what they would see. Bethany would not be breathing, crying, or needing a diaper change. And she never would. The permanence of death, while painfully obvious to adults, can sometimes escape children. It can be important to tell them explicitly that this baby will never be alive again in this world or that they will not grow up and go to school like other children.

Third, Chaplain Ruth made sure they knew there was no one to blame. Emmaline did what she needed to do by getting to the hospital. The staff did everything they should do as well, but the baby still died. She told the kids what a good mother Emmaline was. Adults sometimes ask "Why?" after a death, but when children ask "Why?" it is always concrete. What we mean is that children aren't asking an existential question. They want to know what events or actions led to this tragedy. So, the chaplain needed to explain that no one did anything wrong.

Fourth and finally, Chaplain Ruth set the children up for success by telling them how cute baby Bethany was. "Just wait till you see her little nose," she said. By doing this, she allowed the kids to treasure the baby, not just feel sad about the baby. From there, the kids took over. Their honest emotions and questions–"Can you take off her hat?"–caused Emmaline to crack her first smile.

Sesame Street, the PBS educational children's television series, has aired some shows about death and grief.[2] We encourage you to visit the site in the endnote and watch how these sketches display the best ways to help kids, especially toddlers, understand death. In each of the episodes, when the adult characters discuss death with the children they model the above four behaviors, plus one more. They also communicate the message, "I am here for you." Children need to know that the adults in their lives will be there for them when they need to talk.

In a humorous but realistic scene, Elmo (a preschool character who is a staple of the series) discusses his uncle's death with his father. Elmo's dad exhibits this last behavior as he somewhat nervously tells Elmo that he can ask him any questions he has about death. When Elmo says that he does have one question, his dad looks a little panicked but squares his shoulders for Elmo's difficult question about death and dying. Then Elmo asks if he can take his kite to the park when they go to play. Elmo's dad is relieved that the question is simple to answer. Children often oscillate more quickly than adults between deep questions of grief and mundane, childlike questions about everyday topics. As adults, we need to use age-appropriate techniques with children who are in grief. We communicate support with openness and honesty and allow them to respond individually. We recognize they will sometimes rotate quickly between a range of emotions. We prepare them for the experience by using concrete and specific terms. Talking with kids about death and grief is never easy. But if we use these tools, we can help the little people in our lives.

Notes

1. Thank you to Kathy and Tim Hardin and Bob and Melinda Sexton for allowing me to join you in your grief.

2. https://www.sesamestreet.org/toolkits/grief/

Lori's Story

"I've been through hell and back," Lori said quietly to herself before she sent the article to her publisher, "and I've lived to tell about it."

When Lori was a little girl, her parents sometimes let her stay the night at her grandmother's apartment. Lori loved her times with grandma. She was a kind old woman with a closet full of toys. Lori played for hours, laying on her belly on grandma's shag carpet. Sometimes grandma laid on her belly, too. The two were good friends.

A small wooden sign hung on the wall in her grandmother's cozy bathroom. There was a drawing of a little girl, about Lori's age. She was wearing blue jeans and a yellow sweater, and her arms were wrapped tight around herself. Her eyes were squeezed closed, and she was grinning from ear to ear. She was giving herself a big hug. Below the girl were three words–*You're Worth It!*

Lori felt welcomed and loved at Grandma's. She felt like that little girl. She was worth it. One Saturday night, Lori slept over at Grandma's. While she brushed her teeth, she looked at the sign. It made her feel safe.

Sadly, it was the last time Lori would feel safe for a very long time. Lori's *hell* began later that night.

After Lori went to sleep at grandma's apartment,

her parents were in a horrible car accident. Her dad was driving as they returned home from a nice dinner. The roads were wet. They rounded a curve and a large cargo truck was coming their way on the other side of the road. The head-on collision was devastating. Tragically, Lori's mother was killed instantly, and her dad was badly injured. Lori can still remember waking up early the next morning. Wearing her flannel pajamas, she stepped into her grandmother's family room. Grandma sat on the couch, tears brimming in her eyes. She patted the seat next to her. As Lori sat down, grandma wrapped her arms around Lori and gave her the news.

At the funeral, Lori's dad leaned over the casket, sobbing uncontrollably. Her little heart broke for him.

Lori stayed with her grandma for a few weeks while her dad recovered physically, although he was never quite the same. Her grandmother was always loving and open with Lori, even through that tragedy. On the contrary, her dad was severely withdrawn. He didn't want to talk about what happened, so they never did. They didn't talk about mom. They didn't talk about how dad was doing and certainly didn't discuss how Lori was handling the tragic loss of her mother. In the months that followed, her dad plunged himself into his work. He started drinking more. His relationship with Lori became tense and hurtful.

Many years later, Lori realized that her dad was severely depressed following the accident. His coping mechanism was alcohol. That wasn't good, because he was mean when he was drunk. He blamed himself for the car accident, and secretly hated himself. He took his self-loathing out on Lori. He felt worthless, and he made Lori feel worthless, too. She never did anything good enough to make him happy, even though all she wanted to do was please him. In the years following her mother's death, Lori worked hard at home and school, trying to earn his approval.

Even when Lori's dad wasn't drunk, he called her demeaning names. His favorite was "small fry". It wasn't the worst name he called her, but it hurt Lori just the same. It made her feel unimportant and ignored. It made her feel like her grief didn't matter. Like she didn't matter. Lori's good grades and perfect behavior didn't lessen her dad's contempt for her. His unresolved grief and guilt manifested in the way he treated his little girl. Lori, like many children of alcoholic and abusive parents, learned to ignore her grief, pain, and needs. She also ignored her unique character traits and talents. That is until she no longer could.

In high school, Lori wrote a tender short story for a competition in her creative writing class. The fictional characters were all based on food items; a burger, a soda, and a small fry. The story creatively chronicled the trauma the fries experienced when they were lowered into the fryer. They were terrified and overwhelmed with pain. Once cooked, they were tossed onto a tray, overlooked, and slathered in ketchup. As they were consumed, they asked the question, "Did I even matter?"

The story was poignant and touching, full of symbolism from Lori's own life. It got the attention of her teacher and the committee deciding the winner of the competition. The day Lori was awarded first prize, the school made a copy of her story available for all the other students. She was horrified when everyone began reading her story. She braced for ridicule from her classmates. To Lori's amazement, many people liked the story. The number of students who seemed *touched* by the story was very meaningful to her.

A year later, when Lori was seventeen-years-old, her dad's untreated depression reached its climax. Tragically, he died by suicide. Lori was numb at his funeral. She was sad that he died but sadder that her mom died ten years before. Grief over her mom was still just beneath the surface of her heart.

After her dad's death, Lori moved in with her grandma. That was the first time Lori had felt truly safe since she was a small child, since the night her mother died. Grandma spoke often and openly about her son and daughter-in-law, Lori's parents. Pictures of both of them were always on display around the apartment. Lori didn't always open up to

Grandma about her grief, but she found comfort in writing stories and poetry in her journals.

+++

As an adult, Lori became an accomplished writer. Every job she held included writing in one way or another. She also kept personal journals and created her own stories. Often her stories were sad tales of children in desperate situations, feeling undervalued and unloved. Everyone marveled at her talents, but she thought they were just being nice. She was her own worst critic and was never happy with anything she did-writing or otherwise.

Lori met Jeff through a friend, and they started dating right away. Jeff had a big personality, especially in contrast to Lori. A couple of years later, Jeff and Lori got married and shortly after started a family. They had two daughters in two years. Both pregnancies went smoothly and the girls were a delight.

Jeff and Lori's marriage was rocky from the start. When Lori's grandmother first met Jeff, she was worried. He reminded her of Lori's dad, her son. Instead of seeing Lori as a wonderful, creative person, Jeff made fun of her for being too sensitive and getting lost in her work. He seemed a bit angry, insecure, and liked to drink, as well.

When the girls were nine and eleven years old, the family was surprised to learn that Lori was pregnant with a third child. Lori was thrilled with the idea of another baby. She loved it when her girls were newborns. The skills she developed as a child found a healthy expression when she became a mother. She always prioritized her dad's needs over her own. Now, she had people who naturally needed her. She loved dressing them, toting them around, even feeding them in the middle of the night. Everything about them was so precious and simple. As they got older and gained a bit of independence, Lori pined for the days when they were tiny and helpless with her at home. The girls were with her at the appointment when they found out their wishes had come true-they were having a little boy. They weren't even home yet when the name Benjamin was mentioned. The name felt right to Lori. Lori's grandmother had a stillborn baby a couple of years before Lori's dad was born. She named her baby, Lori's uncle, Benjamin.

"Benjamin," she whispered to herself in the garage after the girls hopped out of the car.

When Lori was young she always wanted a large family. She didn't like growing up as an only child, especially after her mom died. But, she accepted that this would be her last pregnancy. Jeff held obvious angst about the topic of parenting in general. He and the girls were somewhat close when they were little, but Jeff worked even more now and could not always be bothered with family concerns. Distance between him and the girls grew even before everything that happened.

Lori tried to compensate. She even quietly

resigned from a job she loved at a small local company where she served as a director of marketing and communications. She started freelance writing so she could be at home when the girls got off the bus after school, run them to appointments, and generally, take care of everything at home. She imagined Jeff would be happy that she was covering all the bases so he could work long hours and do little when he was home. Unfortunately, he was more concerned that she kept making as much money as she had before.

Freelance writing paid pretty well, and Lori's talents were put to good use. She mostly wrote articles for magazines, either online or in print. The topics were decided for her by the publisher. Then Lori would do some research and wrote something that met the needs of the magazine. Her articles were always well received, and many readers expressed appreciation. Although Lori never wrote from a personal perspective, she still kept her journal. It was filled with personal thoughts and ideas for writing projects from her perspective. She never shared it with anyone-it was far too personal.

Lori was alone when she found out about Benjamin's health problems. The doctor called after her 18-week ultrasound and asked her to come in the next day and bring Jeff. But Jeff was out of town for a work trip again, so Lori was the only one in the room when she got the news that changed everything. She felt like the small fry about to be lowered into the fryer.

Looking back, Lori can't remember much about that appointment, although she remembers the devastating impact. When her doctor first said the word "anomaly", Lori's heart broke to pieces.

Benjamin had a genetic problem.

The problem was not fixable. The only question, the doctor explained, was whether Benjamin would die in her womb or during delivery.

Laden with the worst heartbreak of her life, Lori drove to the bus stop to pick up the girls. She tried to hide her tears, but she could not. By the time they parked in the garage, Lori told them what her doctor said.

"It's Benjamin. The doctor says there's a problem. He has a condition that. It's going to make it really hard for him to live outside of my body. Girls, he might not make it. He might not be born alive."

The girls dropped their backpacks and lunchboxes and wrapped their arms around their mom. They all cried for a long time. Lori felt a little proud that she had been forthright with the girls about her feelings and proud of the compassion and honest emotion they displayed.

Then she called Jeff.

"What is it, honey? I've got another meeting in five minutes." Jeff held a demanding job.

"I just got back from the appointment." Lori was trying to be strong for him. She knew this would be hard to process while he was in the middle of a workday.

"What appointment?" Like usual, Jeff wasn't fully engaged.

"Jeff, my OB appointment, the one they called about yesterday?" Lori was upset, but not surprised.

"Oh yes, I'm sorry. Everything okay?"

Lori started to cry again. "No, Jeff. Benjamin is not okay."

But before she could go on, Jeff said, "Honey, sorry, hold on a minute, I'm having a hard time hearing you. Can I call you back after this meeting?"

"Sure. That's fine." Lori lied to cover her feelings again.

She also wasn't surprised when he forgot to call back after the meeting. It was late that evening before she gave him the news. He sat in stunned silence on the phone.

When he finally spoke, Lori wished he hadn't.

"Maybe it's for the best, Lori. We've got a lot going on. We probably don't have any business bringing another child into the world. Your career is taking off, and work is getting busier and busier for me. The girls are getting older and have more responsibilities. Who knows, maybe we'll be glad this happened."

As Lori sat on their king-sized bed, alone and on the phone, with a perfectly round little belly under her shirt, she thought, "How could I ever be glad that something like this happened?"

Now she sat in stunned silence on the phone until Jeff was too uncomfortable to stay on the line.

"We'll talk about it tomorrow when I get home. Good night, Lori." He hung up before she could say another word.

Lori's heart, once again, was relegated to her journal as her words poured out in one painfully candid sentence after another. She wrote until she was exhausted, and her journal laid open in her bed all night.

+++

Lori's doctor gave her a Doppler device so she could listen for Benjamin's heartbeat at home. Her girls were thrilled and wanted to listen to their brother. But Lori said no. She was afraid. If the one time she let the girls listen was the time Benjamin had no heartbeat, how would they react? How would she react?

Lori's emotions became more and more intense. She felt deeply sad as she anticipated Benjamin's death. She despaired. She stopped talking about Benjamin with the girls. She never started talking about him with Jeff. She tried to maintain her usual activities, but the burden of Benjamin's impending life, birth, and possible death was becoming too much to bear.

Sadly, Benjamin died. Before he was born, and before Lori was full term, he died in Lori's womb. Lori went to the hospital when she could not find his heartbeat. There, the nurses confirmed her fears. Just like she had lost her mom, then her dad, now she had lost Benjamin, too.

One of the cruelest realities of Lori's situation was that she was far enough along that she had to deliver Benjamin in a birthing center. She had to deliver a dead baby, a baby she knew was dead before she even donned her patient wristband and gown, on a unit where moms were having live babies all around her. What's worse was that since her pregnancy wasn't complete, her body was slower to respond to the medicine she was given to induce labor. So, labor was long and hard. The girls were at a friend's house. Jeff was at the hospital. He tried to be helpful, but he failed. The nurses took good care of her physically but didn't connect with her much emotionally.

Lori felt like she couldn't do it. She couldn't make it through labor. She couldn't hold a dead baby. Could she even look at Benjamin, the baby she wanted so badly? She knew he would be so small, and his health issues might make him harder to look at. She accepted all the pain medication she could, and she desperately wanted it all to be over. She just wanted this nightmare to end.

Once Benjamin was born, Lori snapped. What she experienced was not exactly grief or sadness, although that was certainly part of it. But her grief mixed with loneliness, confusion, and, most of all, panic. After saying very little for most of her hospital stay, immediately after his delivery, she began to shriek.

"Benjamin! Benjamin!" She wailed. "My baby! Why? Why? Benjamin! Benjamin!"

A nurse, cut the cord and cleaned Benjamin a little bit. She asked Jeff if he thought it was a good idea for Lori to hold Benjamin. Jeff made the mistake of looking into Benjamin's face. He was shocked. He half expected to see something that didn't look quite human. But Benjamin looked like... a baby. He was small, of course, but other than that he looked like the girls when they were born.

Jeff looked away quickly, back to the nurse. Then he looked at Lori, leaning over the bed, sobbing uncontrollably.

"I think you'd just better get him out of here. I'll try to calm her down." He said, without consulting Lori.

But as the nurse started for the door, Lori's eyes shot open.

"Where are you going? Where are you taking my baby?" She yelled.

"Honey, they're going to take him out for a little bit so you can calm down," Jeff said in a patronizing tone.

Sadly, Lori was too tired to fight, and her mind was blurred and hazy. Even in her fog, she knew Jeff would not stay in the room with her much longer, and she would have an opportunity to hold Benjamin. So, she didn't complain, she just waited.

Later that night, for two hours, Lori held her baby boy. Two hours. That's all she got.

The girls never came to the hospital. Jeff didn't want to have a funeral, but Lori rallied the strength to insist on it. At the funeral, the casket was closed. So, the girls never even laid eyes on their brother. They were heartbroken, angry, and confused. Lori couldn't bring herself to give them much comfort.

Lori oscillated between numbness and total hysteria. At the graveside service, she fell to her knees and draped her body over Benjamin's tiny casket. Less than a week postpartum, her body and mind broke completely. She had to be lifted into the car by Jeff and others.

+++

Lori and Jeff didn't talk much in the months following Benjamin's funeral. They were like ships passing. Jeff's boss at work told him to take a few bereavement days off, but Jeff only took two days, then assured his boss he was fine and plunged back into work. Even more sadly, Lori and the girls started to drift apart. Lori sometimes forgot to pick them up from the bus stop, and they walked home. She tried to ask them about their school days, but her sadness was so paralyzing.

Lori felt guilty about not letting the girls come up to the hospital. They complained to her about it. They said she "ruined everything". They blamed her for Benjamin's death and for keeping them from being able to meet their baby brother. Lori accepted that it was, indeed, all her fault.

She tried to get back to her work but kept missing deadlines. That wasn't like her. So, a couple of her colleagues messaged her to see if she was doing okay. She wrote them back, oversharing about Benjamin's death, the trauma she felt, her distance from Jeff and the girls, and confessed that she was having a hard time putting one foot in front of another.

One colleague, a person she considered a friend, wrote her back right away. She told her she needed to pick herself up, forget about all this, be strong, and move on. Lori was home alone when she read her message. That was good because she screamed at the screen in an outburst she could not control. How could she *move on*?

Another colleague was a woman who sent a lot of work Lori's way over the years. She was extremely wealthy and successful at leading her company. Lori always wished she could be more like Louise. She was so confident and put-together. She told Lori how sorry she was to hear all this. She pledged to keep in touch through the days ahead, sent her several links to online support groups, and articles. Lori was too numb to be touched by the gesture, but she was surprised by the last resource. It was an online test, a test for depression symptoms.

She clicked the link.

On her screen she saw questions like:

How often do you feel helpless?

Lori checked "Always".

How often do you feel you have lost interest in things and activities that used to interest you?

Again, "Always".

How often do you feel overwhelmed?

"Always".

How often do you feel optimistic?

"Rarely".

When she had finished the short quiz, the automated result on her screen shocked her. It shouldn't have, but it did. The test revealed that she was experiencing symptoms of severe depression. It described depression as interfering with her tasks in everyday life. That made her think of the deadlines she had missed for work. The results also indicated that severe depression was likely interfering with her relationships with others. She knew things were not good between her and Jeff. She could blame a lot of that on him. Then she thought about her girls. They were just kids. She could not blame them for their crumbling relationship. The test results explained that while an online test could not provide a diagnosis, it may indicate that she needed to get some help. A phone number was listed to find facilities, counselors, and help nearby. Lori saved the number but didn't make the call.

+++

"I think I'm depressed," Lori told Jeff flatly one evening after the girls had gone to bed.

"Ya think?" Jeff replied callously as he scrolled through emails on his phone, leaning against the kitchen counter.

"Yeah, Jeff, I do." It was hard for Lori to admit her own needs, and Jeff wasn't making it any easier. "I think I need to get some help."

Jeff huffed and said, "I think you need to forget about it and move on."

Lori could tell he had wanted to say that for a long time. She clenched her teeth.

"You mean forget about *him*?" Lori said.

"What?"

"Don't you mean I need to forget about *him*? To forget about Benjamin?" Lori surprised herself with this brief act of defiance towards Jeff.

"Well, it sure as hell isn't doing any good sitting around here and remembering him, is it, Lori? You can barely get out of bed, the girls are fending for themselves, and you're losing work and losing money right and left."

Lori's moment of standing up for herself was over as quickly as it started. Jeff was right, of course. Lori's life was a mess. She knew it, and could not deny his accusations.

But Jeff was also wrong. Lori wished she could remember Benjamin *more*, not less. In fact, she decided, she was going to visit his grave for the first time since the funeral. She thought about the grave day and night. She would visit him tomorrow.

+++

Lori got up and dressed the next morning. That was a big deal because she sometimes stayed in bed until the girls had been at school for a couple of hours. That day, though, she was on a mission. Lori was heading to Benjamin's grave for the first time since she was pulled off his casket after the funeral. She needed to do this, for herself. She thought about her grandma's pictures of her parents. She knew there was a better way to remember loved ones, and she wanted to discover it.

In the garage, she started the car. But before she could put the car into gear, her wild mind started spinning. Why did Benjamin have to die? Why couldn't she keep him alive? Why couldn't she be a good mom? Why couldn't she be the wife Jeff needed, and why couldn't she bring herself to just do her work on time? Why couldn't she be a caring mom to her girls? Why couldn't she keep her dad from being depressed and choosing suicide?

What is wrong with me? This question started to dominate Lori's mind. Irrational tears started flowing down her cheeks as she forced herself to drive. She navigated in the direction of the cemetery, but now she knew she couldn't go there. Her mind was out of control. The darkness of her pain and sadness took over, and she began thinking terrible thoughts–thoughts about ending *her own* life. Driving faster, she was about to steer her car into oncoming traffic. A large cargo truck was coming her way on the other side of the street. Surely she could just... But she didn't. Thoughts of death consumed her. She wondered if she could simply join Benjamin. She wondered if Jeff and the girls would be better off without her. A part of her knew this was crazy, but she could not control her thoughts. She knew she needed help. Because of that little online test, she knew she had the right label for what was happening inside of her. She was severely depressed. She needed help, fast. Could she admit she needed help? Could she let her hurts and grief show to another person? If so, who?

That's when she noticed a big blue sign with a large white "H" and an arrow.

That's it. Lori thought. *I need Help.*

It was hard to explain why she was admitting herself to the emergency department. Thankfully, as a nurse covered intake questions, she asked, "Have you had thoughts of harming yourself?"

"Yes," Lori said simply and bit her lip. How could she deny it? She had those thoughts immediately before coming to the hospital.

Lori's racing mind calmed a bit as she saw one professional after another. Eventually, she was taken to a specialized local facility where she met more staff. They treated her with kindness and respect, something she had not experienced at home in a long time, not since she lived with her grandma anyway.

During her initial session with a counselor, she was asked about any traumatic events in her life recently. She stared at the ground. Tears bubbled and then burst.

"Benjamin!" She shrieked. "My baby!"

The counselor comforted her and let her cry, then asked her to share the story about Benjamin.

Sadly, Lori wasn't very practiced at talking about Benjamin out loud. Jeff just wanted to forget about it. She kept her feelings from the girls. She overshared with some colleagues, but even that was done digitally, not face to face. She hacked through telling the whole story, punctuated with self-shame statements about being a failure in so many ways.

"I couldn't even drive myself to his grave today," Lori admitted as a final defeat.

The counselor was caring and thoughtful and knew better than to attempt too much during their first meeting.

"Lori, you have experienced a traumatic event. Your baby died. It's normal to feel sad and isolated like you lost something precious to you. Because *you did*."

Lori's brief stay at that facility was focused on helping her to be safe. She went on some temporary medications, was given some coping tools, and follow-up appointments with the counselor. When she got home, the girls wrapped their arms around

Lori like they did the day she told them that Benjamin might not be born alive. Jeff forced an awkward hug that made Lori feel like a child.

Lori told Jeff about the medications and the counseling appointments.

"How much is all that going to cost?" Jeff demanded.

"I don't know, Jeff. I'm sorry to be a burden." Just being around Jeff for twenty minutes reinforced Lori's shame that sent her to the hospital in the first place. She felt like she was seven years old again and living with her dad. If she wasn't utterly convinced how necessary this help was, she would have abandoned the plan immediately.

+++

Nothing was magically better after Lori's admission to the behavioral health unit, but she did feel a bit safer. Having a follow-up plan made her feel like she might have a way out of the darkness.

Over the next few months, Lori saw the counselor regularly. In one session she mentioned that journaling was her primary way of coping with life.

"Did Benjamin's death make you stop writing in your journal?" The counselor asked. Lori liked that she always used Benjamin's name.

"Oh no," Lori grinned. "I started writing even more. That's my safe place."

"Would you mind bringing your journals to our next appointment?" The counselor asked.

Lori had grown to trust her counselor, so she

brought her journals to with her the next time they met. The counselor handled them with care, like they were highly valuable, as she started reading Lori's writing. She sniffled. She wiped her tears. Then she laughed a little. After a few minutes of silence, she closed the journals and looked up at Lori with a smile.

"Your voice," she leaned forward as she paused. "Your voice is so valuable, Lori. I think your story needs to be heard."

The counselor cleared her throat and said, "I don't usually do this, but I want to tell you my own story. I won't drag it out, but I think you need to know. When my husband Gary and I were newly married, nearly forty years ago now, I got pregnant for the first time. Six weeks later, I miscarried. I lost that baby. Back then we didn't talk about these things much. I went back to work a few days later. Gary was sweet, but he didn't know how to help me. We never really talked about it. That Christmas, Gary bought me a puppy. I guess he figured that might help. Years later, when I was becoming a counselor, we had to start talking about the baby we lost. Do you know what, Lori? The pain was still there, still very real. Passing all those years in silence didn't fix anything. It just compacted the pain, stuffed it down so far that it took time to get it loosened up. To be honest, we are still working through it."

"What I am telling you, Lori is that when it comes to miscarriage and stillbirth as we have experienced, silence is the enemy. We can't begin to imagine how many moms are going through this pain and sadness. They might be feeling very alone and isolated like they are the only ones facing this grief. Lori, I know that part of my purpose on this earth is to do *this*. To sit here with wonderful people like you and offer a listening ear and some advice that might help. I think," she carefully handed the journals back to Lori, "I think part of your purpose is to *write* about the grief that miscarriage and stillbirth can bring."

Lori hardly blinked while she listened. The counselor repeated what she said before, "Lori, your voice is valuable. You are valuable. Benjamin is precious. And I think you need to share your personal story. You have such a gift, and you might be able to help a lot of people."

+++

As Lori drove home, she felt torn in two. When her counselor talked about using her voice, something came alive inside of her. Although she didn't value her writing as much as others did, she knew she could do it. That was her job, after all. But what her counselor was asking her to do was different. This was personal. She never thought about her journals as something that might be worth sharing. How could she share herself with the world when she wasn't even talking with the three people who shared her home?

She thought about sharing some of her words with Jeff. Anger flashed in her mind.

"He doesn't deserve it." She said out loud. She started to see what her grandma saw from the beginning. Jeff never saw value in Lori. Why would he start now?

Immediately she thought about her girls.

She held no anger toward them. They were her sweet children. Her heart swelled as she thought about how hard all this had been on them. For over a year since Benjamin's death, she was so depressed herself that she could barely think about them. When they were infants she loved making them her top priority. But depression had robbed her of that closeness.

When she got home, the girls were having their after-school snacks, backpacks, and papers strewn around the kitchen. Lori felt like a stranger as she walked in and sat down, one of her journals tucked under her arm.

She tried to make small talk about their days at school, but it went nowhere. She wanted to apologize. She wanted to tell them how much she missed Benjamin, and that she knew they did, too. She wanted to hold them, love them, and reconnect. All her feelings were simmering just below the surface as the girls ate their snacks, then headed to their rooms without saying a word.

That night, Jeff came home earlier than usual.

"I had a counseling appointment today," Lori reported.

"Seriously? How many more do you have?" Jeff was sorting through some mail at the kitchen island.

"I'm not sure, Jeff. I don't think that's how this works. There's not a deadline of when I will be magically healed." Lori's words had an edge that she was quietly proud of. She was not well-practiced at standing up for herself yet.

"Well, that sucks. I think I went into the wrong field. If I got paid per hour what we are paying that freaking counselor, I'd be retired by now." Jeff walked towards the bedroom.

"You could *never* do what she does," Lori said under her breath. She didn't think Jeff would hear her. After all, listening wasn't his strong suit.

"What did you just say?" Jeff looked her in the eye for the first time in weeks.

"Nothing," Lori said.

"You don't think I could sit in a room with people like *you* for an hour and listen to you whine about how hard your life is? Yeah, Lori, I'm sure that's a real challenge." Jeff hated that she was seeing the counselor. "Actually, you know what? You're probably right. After listening to people's petty problems for a week, I'd probably want to kill myself, too."

Lori couldn't take it anymore. Her dad had devalued her as a child. Jeff had heaped shame and embarrassment on her since the beginning of their marriage. She hid her true feelings for so long. But, no more. She was ready to come out of hiding.

Words that had been suppressed inside of her for years finally started to boil over.

"Petty problems, Jeff? How can you stand there and say that giving birth to a stillborn baby is a petty problem? Do you have any idea what that has done to me? I got two hours with my only son. The son I wanted so badly. Did you even notice, Jeff, that his first birthday would have been last month? Of course, you didn't." Lori was only beginning, but Jeff jumped in, trying to maintain control.

"No, Lori, you know why? Because I'm over it. I moved on. Good God, Lori, you've got to get over it. You've got to forget about it!" Jeff shouted with a red face.

"You….mean….*him*! He has a name. You probably don't even remember it because of how hard you've worked to forget it. To forget him. Let me give you a reality check, Jeff. I will *never* forget Benjamin. Never. He's my son. My only boy. I wanted him. I want him now. I miss him. I wish he was here. I wish I was chasing him around the house as he toddles from one room to the next. I wish I was putting him down for a nap and hustling down to the basement to write my next article. I wish I was cramming his chubby feet into cute little shoes. I wish I was snapping overalls on his round little shoulders. I wish I was changing his diapers, feeding him toddler foods, and strapping him into his car seat. I wish our girls were playing with him, showing him off to their friends, and getting irritated when he gets into their things. I wish, I wish that bedroom upstairs where his bed is still set up had a pint-sized occupant that plays with balls and cars. I wish I was visiting his pediatrician instead of his grave. His daycare instead of a counselor. Scheduling playdates instead of support groups. I'm never going to move on, Jeff! I'm never going to forget about Benjamin. I'm never going to get over it. To get over him. So, screw you, Jeff!"

As Jeff stormed out of the house, Lori crumpled in the middle of the kitchen floor. The sound of Jeff's car speeding away from the house was followed by quiet footsteps coming down the stairs. She could not lift her head, but when she felt two sets of young arms wrap around her, she felt more valued and loved than she had in a long time.

"I'm so sorry, girls," Lori said as she sat up, realizing that they were both crying, too.

But the girls would not accept her apology, because they loved what she said. They hadn't heard her talk like this in a long time. They realized how much their mom was hurting, and it allowed them to be honest with her about their sadness. They both called her *Mommy* over and over. They all three said Benjamin's name more times than they could count. They talked about what they were missing about him, and how special he is. Lori kissed the tears off their cheeks. They cried, laughed, and apologized until they all realized how hungry they were.

"How about I make some burgers?" Lori asked.

"Benjamin burgers," said the younger sister.

Lori laughed and nodded. "I do have a feeling that he would have had a big appetite and loved burgers. So, yes, let's have burgers in honor of Benjamin. We will imagine what it would have been like to eat with Benjamin pulled up in his high chair, making a mess of ketchup and applesauce. We'll think about how many sippy cups we would have filled every day over the last year. And," she put an arm on each girl's shoulders, "we won't apologize to anyone."

+++

"So, things are going a *lot* better with the girls," Lori told her counselor at her next appointment. "Jeff, on the other hand... He's just done. He's done with Benjamin. He's done with coming home after work. He's done with the girls. He's done with me. I expect to get papers from his lawyer any day. It makes me sad, but I can't keep ignoring my feelings any longer. When I ignore my feelings and my needs, I'm ignoring my daughters' feelings, too. And that's just not okay anymore."

Lori was right. Just a few weeks after the fight that sparked Lori's wildfire, the fight where Lori finally stood up for herself, her girls, and Benjamin, she got divorce papers in the mail.

She sat the girls down immediately. They had talked about this possibility. They weren't any more surprised than Lori. The girls were older now and hadn't been close with Jeff in a long time. Because of that, their sense of loss over their dad was less than their grief over their brother. It was sad, but Lori and the girls talked it out and processed all the changes together. Lori's caring nature was shining through again. In turn, the girls also helped her along this new journey.

+++

One day, as Lori was finishing a writing piece for Louise, her colleague who had referred her to the online test for depression symptoms, her phone rang. It was the principal of the school her girls attended. He told her that Lori's oldest daughter, Elyse, was in his office and he wondered if Lori could come to the school. She felt panicked and came right away.

In the principal's office, Lori learned that her daughter had spoken to her English class about Benjamin's death. The assignment was to tell a story about something that happened in your life that changed who you are. So, she talked about her brother. During the presentation, she shed some tears. Everyone clapped and her teacher handed out tissues. However, a few hours later, Elyse was in gym class when a troublemaking boy made fun of her for being so sensitive. He said that she was a crybaby. He didn't think Elyse would hear him, but after so many years of living with her dad, her hearing was perfectly tuned for hurtful comments.

So, she heard him immediately. Unlike Lori, Elyse would not tolerate anyone putting her down. So, her response to this boy led her to the principal's office.

When Lori arrived, Elyse was still crying as the principal told the story.

"So, ma'am, Elyse hit the boy," the principal explained.

"What?" Lori was stunned.

"Right in the eye." The principal pointed to his eye, just to be clear.

"Okay."

At that very moment, on the other side of a large window, the nurse's office door opened and out walked a boy in eighth grade, about six inches taller than Elyse and fifty pounds heavier. His hair was unkempt and Lori could tell he had been crying. She thought his right eye might have been a little swollen.

Lori's own wide eyes came back to Elyse. Then the principal.

She knew what the principal wanted to hear. "Well, violence is certainly not acceptable in school. Thank you so much for calling me. Will it be okay if I take Elyse home for the rest of the day?"

"Yes, of course. If there's anything more, I'll be in touch."

On the monitor, the school secretary saw Elyse walk out, arms crossed, and crying. And she saw Lori, arm around Elyse's shoulders, with a slight grin on her face.

"Mom, let me explain," Elyse started, as she got into the car. She was wearing an adorable pair of blue jean overalls with a neon pink t-shirt and white sandals. "He was laughing at me for crying. But sometimes I just have to cry. My little brother died, you know? And that's sad. There's nothing wrong with crying. It's like you say, mom. It doesn't matter who you are, when you are sad, you've got to talk about it, and it's okay if you cry. And if those sad feelings get overwhelming, you've got to get help. I wanted everyone to know that, just in case, you know, just in case they ever have someone die in their lives, or they get depressed. So, when he started laughing at me, it just made me so *angry*. I just had to stop him." Elyse started to cry again. She did not apologize for crying. "So, before I knew it, I hit him. I'm so sorry I did that, mom. Please don't yell at me."

"Well, obviously, violence is not the answer," Lori said, in a voice like she was making a public service announcement. "However, I have a feeling that boy will think twice before putting down someone for crying again. What you did was wrong. But what you were feeling was right." Lori squeezed her hand. "Did you see his eye?"

"Not really. Was it bad?"

"It was a little puffy, I think."

Both of them laughed a bit. Then Lori drove Elyse to her favorite restaurant and ordered her favorite milkshake. They held hands in the car and talked about Benjamin, about dad not being around anymore, about high school next year, and Lori made a confession. She told Elyse she was thinking of writing an article about Benjamin. She was going to say more, but Elyse jumped in.

"You totally should! Mom, who knows how many people are like us? You could really help them. They might be depressed like you were, or just angry like I was. They might need to hear our story. I remember that night when you and dad fought about Benjamin. Your voice was so...noble." It was a strange word to use, but they both felt it was the right word. "More people need to hear *that* voice. It's so valuable."

Lori knew she was right. Her counselor had been saying it for a year or more.

Lori's journals were full of her unvarnished thoughts about Benjamin, her parents, grief, her soul, depression, her disappointments in her marriage, friends, herself, and society in general. Maybe it was time to finally speak out.

+++

A few months later, Lori and Jeff's divorce was final. He did not attempt to feign interest in spending time with the girls, which was fine with Lori. The girls were getting older, and her relationship with them had gone from cold and stifled to warm and enjoyable. It was sad that Jeff was gone, but it was not sad that an unhealthy silence left with him. That silence fueled Lori's depression and her sense of worthlessness.

Once the silence was lifted (about Benjamin, grief, depression, and just about everything else), the house became a welcome refuge. Lori never forgot to get the girls from the bus stop. They cooked dinner together whenever they weren't running from one activity to the next. Lori got over her fear of visiting Benjamin's grave, and she took the girls often. Sometimes it was a sad moment, and they all cried. Other times, they laughed, or sang, or just took a nice walk around the lovely grounds of the cemetery.

One night after a dinner of pancakes, eggs, and breakfast meat, Lori opened up to the girls again. The smell of maple syrup and bacon frying was like a warm blanket laying over each of them.

"I emailed some of my colleagues today," She sipped her coffee and grinned.

"About your special project?" Elyse asked excitedly. That's what they were calling Lori's writing pieces on Benjamin and their experience of losing him.

Lori nodded and smiled.

"And?" The girls asked impatiently.

"Three editors already wrote back. They all want to run it. They're going to have to fight over who gets it first."

The girls were thrilled and proud. They spent the next hour planning topics for Lori's future articles about Benjamin. By the next day, Lori had her first draft done when she picked them up from the bus stop. They hurried home, got their snacks, and Lori read what she had written.

Two hours. That's all I got. Two hours.

My son, Benjamin, was born still. Yet, he was still born. His heart stopped beating before he was born. Life was gone from his little body before it passed through my body, a body that was beginning to feel dead itself. Then, I held him in my arms for two hours.

I told my girls I didn't want them to come to the hospital. A decision for which I am still doing penance, though their tenders hearts have extended forgiveness. The nurses didn't know what to do with me since I wasn't learning to breastfeed, watching him get shots, or trying out his car seat for the trip home.

My husband, the one person in the world whose devastation should have been at least similar to mine, instead only multiplied my pain with his lack of caring, understanding, and openness. He just wanted me to get over it, to get over Benjamin, as quickly as possible. To forget our son and move on with my life and career.

For months, I tried to do what he wanted. I wondered what was wrong with me. Why couldn't I move on? It seemed the rest of the world had moved on. Why couldn't I get back to normal?

Eventually, I had to be honest with myself. I had to admit that I was depressed. It took six months just to admit it to myself, and I still didn't talk with anyone else about it. I stuffed it down deep. It took me two more months to get help, and I only did that after having thoughts of ending my own life.

I felt guilty. Guilty that I had let my baby die. Guilty that I had hurt my girls. I was ashamed that my marriage was falling apart. My life was crumbling around me, and I felt like it was all my fault. I've made my living by writing words. Communicating. But when it came to Benjamin, the only place I could even utter his name was in my journals.

Then, two powerful women inspired me. One was my counselor. What she said rings in my ears every morning when I wake up. Every time my girls climb into my car. Every time I feel depressing thoughts creep back in. Every time I hear of another mom having to say goodbye forever to their child at any age.

She told me, "Your voice must be heard. Your voice matters. You matter."

The second inspirational woman was my own daughter. She cannot and will not tolerate any attempts to belittle our grief over her brother. Her indignation fans my voice into flames.

But my voice can't be heard if I don't speak up.

When I spoke up to my spouse, he closed me off.

When I spoke up to my daughters, they opened their arms to me.

Nearly three years later, it still feels like I'm confessing a sin or admitting a character flaw when I say that I was depressed. But I'm done pretending. I'm done with silence. It's true. My voice needs to be heard. And being depressed doesn't mean I'm worthless. It means I needed help.

Maybe there's someone reading this right now who needs to be hear that you are valuable. You matter. Your heartbreak matters. Your baby matters.

Is it uncomfortable to talk about a miscarriage or a stillbirth? Yes.

Does it do anyone any good to suffer in silence? No.

How much longer must we wait for our silence to be broken?

How much longer must our mothers whose babies died in the silence of the past be ignored?

How much longer will it be acceptable to

simply not know how to talk with moms in grief?

How much longer until we break the silence?

Well, I can tell you one thing. Two hours was not enough with my son.

But three years of silence has been enough. Three years of pretending I'll just be strong and move on. Three years of feeling like my grief is less than the grief of others because no one else got to hold my boy. Three years of minimizing my own needs and ignoring my grief. Three years is enough.

Benjamin may have only been in my arms for two hours. But he is a permanent part of my life.

Benjamin was the smallest person I have ever met. But his impact is larger than I could have imagined, no matter how small he was.

He matters. My daughters matter. I matter.

For my sake, and for your sake, we've got to talk about this.

To the mom who miscarried last week or had a stillbirth last year or fifty years ago; we need your voice, too.

Our voices must be heard. For our own sake. For the sake of our sons and daughters who are gone too soon.

The girls started crying with the first line. They

started clapping after the last line. They hopped up, came around the kitchen table, and wrapped their arms around Lori again.

+++

Lori's colleague, Louise, published Lori's final draft a few months later. Louise was the colleague who sent Lori the online depression symptom quiz. She was more than happy to tackle such a difficult topic, as Lori discovered. She told Lori that when she was a younger woman she had miscarriage after miscarriage. She eventually carried her daughter to full term, and she grew into a fine woman. But years later she still thought often of all those losses, all those babies. Louise knew that the topic needed more conversation, and she also knew that Lori's skill as a communicator would be the perfect prompt for such a conversation.

The morning after the article had been published, Lori walked into her kitchen after taking the girls to school and opened her computer. Lori made her coffee and sat down. What she saw next blew her mind. Her inbox was flooded with messages from one mom after another. Most of the messages thanked her for her honesty, then shared their own story of miscarriage or stillbirth. Some women had lost children decades ago. Others were in the throes of miscarrying as they wrote messages to Lori in response to her article. What was clear was that these moms needed what Lori gave them. She gave them affirmation and a voice. She helped them see that their babies mattered, just like Benjamin. She helped them see that they mattered, a lesson she was still learning about herself.

After Lori read a couple of dozen messages, her phone rang. It was Louise.

"So..." Louise started, then laughed, and paused. "Have you gotten any responses to your article yet?" She was scrolling through the comments online.

"Lori," Louise said, "I know when I am onto something, and we are onto something. I'd like to announce today that we are launching a whole new segment of our magazine, totally dedicated to the topic of miscarriage, stillbirth, and pregnancy loss. I'd like you to take the lead. It will include articles, online forums, Q&A, and live videos. What do you think?"

Lori had success with her writing before. But she hadn't felt this nervous since all her classmates read "Small Fry" in high school. This topic was so personal. Could she share her heart, her mental health concerns, stories about her and the girls, and their grief? More importantly, who was she to try and help so many people with such a difficult need? She felt undeserving. She felt like an impostor.

"What would we call it?" Lori asked.

"Rereading your article this morning, four words jumped out to me: *No Matter How Small*. We can highlight how small Benjamin was, but how much his life means. We can highlight how small your time with him was, but how he's a part of your life forever. We can highlight that this is a topic that gets such little attention even though it's a widespread phenomenon." Louise could feel Lori's anxiety, but she asked again. "Lori, what do you think?"

Lori took a deep breath, glanced at the computer where yet another message from a grieving mom had just appeared.

Lori's mind flashed back to her grandma's house. She was seventeen-years-old again. She remembered her grandma sharing openly about the loss of both of Lori's parents. She remembered how safe she felt with her. She wondered if she could give that gift to people, too. Then she remembered that little plaque in her grandma's apartment. Lori felt like the little girl in that picture again. She felt her grandmother's spirit repeat the words from that frame: *You're Worth It!*

"Lori?" Louise probed.

"Yes."

"You'll do it?" Louise was smiling on the phone.

"Yes. Yes, I will."

+++

A few months, a dozen articles, several Q&As, guest writers, and site development later, Lori was preparing for a live video on *No Matter How Small*. A movement was born out of this platform, and Lori's words and heart shaped it all. She wasn't just sharing her story, she was highlighting other parents, doing research and interviews, and creating online communities of support.

During this particular live video, Lori was addressing one of the most common topics in her new community, the thoughtless comments of others to parents in grief.

Lori sat at her kitchen table with her camera trained on her face. She was always nervous before going live, but once the camera turned on, her passion was contagious. Her authenticity and energy were engaging, which is why her following grew so quickly.

"Has anyone else heard *attachment* comments? People telling you not to be so attached, or that it's good your baby wasn't here for long so you didn't get attached? Did everyone forget about the umbilical cord, people?" Lori's expression was one of humorous confusion. "Remember the placenta? Do you know how I would describe every baby in a mother's womb? I think the word *attached* is pretty appropriate. So, friends, if you feel a little "too attached" to your baby who died, just remember, they really were attached. Quite literally, attached to you. So, it's okay that you still feel attached to them, too."

Moms from all over the world tuned in to Lori's video to find hope and healing–to feel *safe*. One mom watched while folding laundry on the pink love seat in her front room. The late evening sun was fading and the shadow of autumn leaves danced through the large front window. She remembered when Auntie Jean had told her husband something very similar to what Lori described in the video. Jayda heard it many times from the members of her support group over the past few years. Her son, Levi, was two years old and still very much attached. He pulled at Jayda's shirt while she watched Lori's video. As she looked into his big dark eyes, she imagined Amani's brown eyes with long eyelashes, like her own. She wondered if Toby would have ever stood a chance against such a precious daughter. His tree painting hung on the wall nearby, the precious D + A, Daddy loves Amani, carved into the trunk.

Jayda turned her gaze to the painting. "We're still pretty attached to you," Jayda said out loud to Amani. "After all, you're the reason that mommy is taking all these classes to become a counselor. It can be a little exhausting. Waiting tables, chasing you," she said to Levi, "and school on top of it all. But if I can help a few moms and dads as our counselor helped us, it'll all be worth it."

Another mom, in her apartment, but no longer alone, was watching Lori's video in her kitchen. She was cleaning up from the delicious dinner that her husband prepared. Emmaline recalled when her mother came to visit after Baby Bethany died. She had said that same thing. "Thank goodness you didn't have enough time to get attached." Three years later and she could still hear her mom's voice saying hurtful, thoughtless things to her. Her attachment to her full-term, stillborn baby girl had not decreased one bit. Her support group friends were a source of joy and relief for Emmaline in the months and years after Baby Bethany died. And one friend was a source of something more than support. They were having lunch one day when this friend said something very unexpected to Emmaline.

"You need to meet my brother."

"Excuse me?" Emmaline didn't even know she had a brother.

"Yeah, you do. He's a contractor. He works long hours, like you. He needs to get out more, like you. And he eats dinner alone in his apartment a lot, like you. Plus, he's the sweetest guy. He's never been married, and I think he'd make a great dad and husband."

"Well, it sounds like you've got us married already, and we haven't even met!" Emmaline agreed to meet Jarritt just once for dinner. But one dinner turned into another, then another, until Emmaline wasn't eating alone very often anymore.

At the wedding, Emmaline's wedding party was special. Emma Jr. was the flower girl, of course, lovely in a simple white dress. Haley was her maid of honor and prayed over Emmaline in the bride room before the ceremony. Brad did a reading, and there were two bouquets on the stage to remember both Bethanies. Since Emma's dad had died, and she wasn't close to her brother, she asked a special young man to walk her down the aisle.

Micah said, "Well, Auntie Emma, if we could be angry together when my mom and your baby died, I suppose we can be happy together on your wedding day." His grin exposed sweet dimples in his cheeks.

When the pastor asked, "Who gives this woman to be married to this man?" Micah replied, "My mother and I."

His sweet reply didn't make Emmaline cry, but Jarritt was another story. Between seeing Emmaline in her wedding dress, the bouquets, and hearing Micah mention his mom, Jarritt started to cry. Luckily, his best man was prepared with some tissues. He knew Jarritt well. He knew it would happen sooner or later.

On the broadcast of the video, when Lori talked about attachment, Jarritt stood behind Emmaline in their kitchen. He reached down and patted Emmaline's belly, which was growing as the time approached for their son to be born.

"Emmaline," he said with tears in his eyes again, "I don't know if I could feel any more attached to this little guy than I do already. I can't imagine how you felt when you lost Bethany."

Jayda and Toby, with Levi hanging on tight, and Emmaline and Jarritt together in their kitchen, miles apart and yet very much together, heard Lori conclude the episode the same way she always did.

"And remember everyone out there. A person's a person, no matter how small. Good night."

17. Mental Health After Loss

More is being discovered about the mental health toll that miscarriage and stillbirth can take on a woman. You may already be familiar with Postpartum Depression, which can occur in women even after the delivery of a healthy baby. The same experience is possible for a mom whose baby died, of course. However, there are other risks as well.

A recent study revealed that 30% of women displayed symptoms of Post Traumatic Stress Disorder (PTSD) one month after experiencing a miscarriage or ectopic pregnancy.[1] 25% displayed signs of moderate to severe anxiety, and 11% displayed signs of moderate to severe depression, like Lori.

Nine months after the miscarriage, when the rest of the world has gone back to "normal", 18% of women continue to show signs of post-traumatic stress, 17% displayed moderate to severe anxiety, and 6% showed signs of moderate to severe depression.

For us, losing Stephen to miscarriage was certainly the most traumatic event of our lives up to that point. The same could be said for Jayda and Toby and so many others.

For Lori, her lack of support or an outlet to talk about her feelings only magnified the trauma she had experienced. Although simply talking about a traumatic experience isn't always enough to maintain your mental health, an inability to talk about it is certainly a hindrance. As we work with grieving mothers and families every day, from all walks of life, we often find that people just need to tell the story.

After all, how often do you get to tell these stories?

When we speak to groups, we often spend the breaks listening to people's stories about when their mom died, or when they had a stillborn baby, or when their sibling died from cancer. Once they have told us the story, they often thank us for helping them so significantly. They're not just being nice, they really feel we have helped them just because we stood still long enough to listen to them. The formal presentation on death, end of life, grief, finding meaning, etc., gave them the opening they needed to talk about what they had been through. It's almost like there is a magic unknown number of times we need to tell the story before we are "okay". That doesn't mean that we are suddenly unaffected by the experience, it just means our brain is processing the experience.

When it comes to miscarriage and stillbirth, these are hard stories to tell. Finding a safe person or place to discuss your experience with is key to your mental health.

Grief and Trauma

Nearly every parent who loses a child will experience grief. However, trauma can be minimal or overwhelming.

Here are some factors that can add trauma to grief:

1. **Location.** We've known moms who miscarried in the bathroom of a gas station while on a trip far from home. We also know moms whose experience was in a modern hospital, yet they were treated without dignity, to say nothing of how their baby was handled, and those images can stay with the person for the rest of their lives.

2. **Medical complications.** If mom experienced lots of complications (hemorrhaging, infections, abnormal levels of pain, etc.), her grief may have trauma mixed in. Like Jayda, I (Kristen) had to have surgery after our miscarriage. While I wouldn't quite call it traumatic, facing my very first surgery was still pretty terrifying. My surgery was uncomplicated. But it certainly presents the

possibility of a more traumatic experience.

3. **Lack of compassionate care.** While one would think that any mom who is experiencing a loss would garner the most compassionate care imaginable, there are times that the care team or family is so uncomfortable with the situation they avoid it altogether or try to engage as little as possible. When our miscarriage happened, I got a call from the provider after our appointment. He said he was sorry to hear about our *Fetal Demise*. I replied, "You mean the death of our baby?" His insensitivity and use of clinical terms is something that still haunts me all these years later. We wish that was the worst story we have heard about how grieving moms are sometimes treated. Even when the care from a medical team and family is superbly compassionate, grief can still be intense. But when there is a lack of care, that grief can be complicated with added trauma.

4. **Regret.** I find that there are three common regrets for moms. These regrets can be sticky. They can stick with you even when you have tried to grieve well. They can hinder a mother's mental health. They are:

   1. "I didn't get enough time with my baby." This may seem obvious, and it is. But there are ways to maximize your time with baby,

especially if your loss happened later in pregnancy.[2] If you didn't know or weren't provided with these opportunities, it might be something you regret.

2. "I didn't take pictures with my baby." In my experience, many parents initially say they do not want photos, especially if a stillbirth was unexpected and sudden. However, in talking with moms and dads years later, many are so thankful they had professional pictures taken. Those who did not have pictures, good pictures, often regret missing this opportunity. But let me be clear. It should not rest on mom's shoulders to *think* of taking pictures in this traumatic moment. Those around her need to help her make this decision. The shock she is experiencing may keep these thoughts from coming to her mind.

3. "Other important people didn't get to meet my baby." The choice about whether or not to have children, grandparents, friends or others visit the hospital during these difficult moments must be made by each individual. Lori did not let her daughters visit Benjamin in the hospital. Later, she regretted that. Many moms regret not sharing a little time with a few other important people. If it's possible, I recommend having the most important

people in your life share these fleeting moments. It can lessen the trauma you bear because others share your heartbreak. Some regrets are inevitable, but that doesn't mean they don't add to mom's mental burden.

Neither of us is a mental health professional. But it's easy to see that there is an unmet need for many moms (and dads) after a baby dies. Lori got help just in time. If you or someone you know might need the kind of help Lori received, don't wait. A simple online search for the national suicide hotline gives you immediate access to help. If you prefer an online quiz like Lori's, try the UK's National Health Service mood self-assessment.[3]

The bottom line is that losing a baby isn't something to just get over or from which you move on. A woman may suffer significant mental health effects. These effects should not be ignored or overlooked. Even if the impact is not as significant as severe depression and suicidal thoughts, mental health should be taken seriously. Thoughts of self-harm must always be addressed immediately. A general sense of not being yourself could be a more subtle signal that you need help in the form of a therapist or counselor, a clergy person, a support group, or just a caring friend who will listen to you tell the same stories over and over.

Lori clearly experienced depression and thoughts

of hurting herself. She may also have had symptoms of PTSD. When she was admitted to the behavioral health facility and talked with the counselor, remember how she shrieked out Benjamin's name? She did the same thing just after giving birth to him. For six months she had not talked about it or mentally processed this pain. That meant it was as fresh six months later as it was that day in the delivery room. She had a flashback to the most traumatic event of her life. With compassionate listening, some medical intervention, and other tools, her counselor was able to help Lori regain a sense of herself. She was able to integrate her grief into her life—and what a productive life she led!

There is hope.

There is help.

You are not alone.

Notes

1. https://www.ajog.org/article/S0002-9378(19)31369-9/fulltext
2. There are a variety of options for cooling baby so he/she can stay with you longer. Cuddle Cots and Caring Cradles are tools that many hospitals have available.
3. https://www.nhs.uk/conditions/stress-anxiety-depression/mood-self-assessment/

18. Why Doesn't My Partner Understand?

People process grief differently. When the person you are closest to (spouse, significant other, etc.) is processing the loss differently, it can pose a serious challenge.

1. **Internal vs. External.** This could also be called mental vs. verbal. Some people process life verbally, or externally. Others process internally. This doesn't just apply to grief. If your partner processes general life more internally, don't be surprised if he doesn't talk about his grief much. The problem comes when we expect the other person, or even pressure him, to handle his sadness the same way we do. If I like to talk things out and he won't open up, then I could think he is *wrong* or *uncaring*. That may be a totally incorrect assumption. The internal processor may need to tell the verbal processor that they do care and that they are thinking about the baby. They just can't talk about it as much. The verbal person may need to accept that talking about her grief could be draining to her quieter partner. That doesn't mean she can't talk about

it with him, it just means she needs to do so with awareness and sensitivity.

2. **Angry vs. Sad**. Grief can manifest in many forms. I (Kristen) was mostly just sad. Patrick was more angry than sad. I (Patrick) can remember my anger being confusing to Kristen. That could have put a distance between us. But she was gracious and let me feel something she was not feeling.

3. **Visible vs. Hidden.** Opportunities for memory-making are more numerous than ever. Those items might be on display in the home of a grieving family or couple. Pictures might comfort one partner while they disturb the other. Likewise, being public online can be a point of disagreement. One partner may want to post their feelings and experiences while the other prefers to be more private. Finding a balance that honors the feelings of both partners is important.

4. **World changer vs. Let it be.** Some people, after a loss experience, want to change the world for others. We've had parents buy tissues (good tissues, not the hospital variety) to put with bereavement packs. Others have written books, bought critical supplies and bereavement materials, etc. Entire non-profits have grown out of grief. Other parents prefer to focus on finding personal healing, and these efforts may feel like they reopen a wound they

would rather leave alone. Neither feeling is wrong. Recently, I met a lovely couple who had a stillbirth a few years ago. The mother wrote a book, got it illustrated, and was sharing it far and wide. Her husband is a modern cowboy/farmer type. He attended the meeting along with her to talk about the book she wrote, expressed appreciation for the opportunities she had been given and was sweetly supportive. They were quite different. But when she said her goal was to be on major television news channels to tell people about their experience, he just smiled and nodded. When she appears on those shows, he will likely be at her side, still smiling and nodding. They are a great example of how two people can be different—one trying to change the world while the other might prefer to be quieter. But his support of her was obvious, and she wasn't trying to turn him into something he wasn't. She appreciated his unwavering support.

The statistics for how couples usually fair after the death of a child are not encouraging. Lori and Jeff were at odds. She needed to talk about it, and he wasn't interested. She was sad, and he was angry. She needed help, and he wanted to forget about it. Lori and Jeff were already having problems before Benjamin died. When Jeff's mom died, he avoided talking or thinking about it at all costs. He turned to work and alcohol. When Benjamin died, he did the same thing.

His choices came at a cost not only to himself but also to Lori and the girls.

If we can learn one thing from Jeff, it's that trying to ignore loss and grief is a surefire way to be destroyed by it. Lori tried to ignore it in her own way, and it nearly destroyed her. Once her silence was lifted, she started down the road to health and healing. Jeff was unwilling to join her.

Marriages and relationships don't have to suffer because of loss. But they do have to adjust so that each partner has what they need.

19. Fetal Anomalies

Pregnant mothers today know so much more about their unborn babies than in the past. That means that more moms are like Lori–they know ahead of time when the baby has health problems or differences. Some of those anomalies mean that life after birth is very unlikely for the baby. A range of Trisomy disorders (genetic), anencephaly (underdeveloped brain and lack of adequate skull bones), or major organ concerns like a lack of kidneys, heart malformations, etc., usually mean that life outside of the womb will be impossible.

Moms who learn about such serious concerns, sometimes referred to as "incompatible with life", can choose to carry their baby to term, as long as the baby lives, or they can choose early induction, even while the baby has a heartbeat. This is not an easy decision and is always accompanied by advanced medical care, lots of conversations, and conclusive testing.

It's hard to think of an upside to these situations, but here are some bits of help and supports, whichever choice mom makes:

1. **Perinatal Palliative Care.** Palliative care is often reserved for adults nearing the end of life. It's not hospice care, although the two

often work together. Palliative care means caring for a person whose medical situation is not curable. It means making them comfortable and helping them to enjoy the parts of life that are important to them while managing whatever their medical situation might be. Palliative care can be a good option for moms whose babies are unlikely to survive after birth. Perinatal palliative care helps parents embrace whatever life their baby might be able to have before and after birth.

2. **Birth planning.** Many moms do birth planning. For a woman who knows her baby is unlikely to survive, birth planning can be important. She can decide ahead of time not only what medical interventions she wants, but also which ones she declines. She can plan who she wants to be involved and how she wants to connect with her baby during the short time she will have.

3. **Memory making.** These difficult situations present a unique opportunity. Parents can make the most of the time while the baby is still alive in utero. We've known parents who have scheduled photoshoots, taken the baby to special places or to visit special people, and done other anticipated activities together. Sometimes, due to the pain involved in expecting the baby's death, mom can't engage in these activities. Other times, she sees the

window of time between diagnosis and delivery as her best opportunity to make memories with her baby.

4. **Organ donation.** For a slim percentage of these babies, organ donation can be an option. Your doctor and state-sanctioned organ procurement organization can determine eligibility.

5. **Bereavement doulas.** There is a growing field of bereavement doulas, midwives, counselors, and other helpers. If a woman knows she is giving birth to a baby with significant anomalies, she could contact one of these professionals for help.

20. The Church

We have both been in church our whole lives. We both grew up in Roman Catholic Churches and spent our adult lives mostly in Protestant, evangelical churches. For seventeen years, Patrick worked in churches as an intern, youth minister, associate minister, and senior pastor. He is an ordained minister. Currently, he serves as the Director of Chaplaincy for a large health system, Parkview Health, in Indiana. The position has some religious duties but isn't associated with one particular church. We have years of experience in various churches. The church can be the soft and supportive place that people in grief need. Or not.

There are a few major hurdles that the church stumbles over when trying to help people in grief.

- **Religious rites and rules.** Sometimes theology doesn't know how to respond to unexpected circumstances. Church doctrine, like state and federal laws, are established for the expected situation. Miscarriage and stillbirth are unexpected. Theology is often very cut and dry about life and death. When I (Patrick) was interviewed to be a chaplain, I was asked how I would respond to a baptismal request for a baby who had died. That reminded me of an unexpected circumstance our own family had faced years before. Kristen's sister delivered her daughter, Kamille, stillborn at twenty-four weeks. The family called in their pastor. He performed a beautiful baptismal service at the bedside. There are many experiences in life that Kami has missed. However, with Pastor Jim's help, she did not miss this important sacrament. He didn't let his theology of the *expected* keep him from blessing those experiencing the *unexpected*. So, when I was asked the question about baptism during my interview, I cried, remembering Kami's baptism. We wish the world was full of Pastor Jims. However, we've heard the heartbreak and confusion of families in *unexpected* situations too many times to fail to mention it here. In the church, we can often be ensnared with our theology of the expected.

- **Evangelical triumphalism.** We are in an era of win-at-all-costs Christianity. In an evangelical church you will often hear things like, "God never loses", "All things work together for our good", or other sentiments that seem to make God and Christians out to be the automatic winners in any given situation. There's a very popular song currently whose refrain repeats "I'm gonna see a victory." It's what I call Phase Two thinking in my book, *How to Talk with Sick, Dying, and Grieving People*. In this religious context, we don't know what to do with grief. It feels like a loss (duh!), which runs counter to everything we think Christianity is about. Because of this, grieving and hurting people get lost in the shuffle. And I'm sorry about that.

- **Religious platitudes.** In *How to Find Meaning in Your Life Before it Ends*, I discuss the damaging nature of platitudes in the lives of the grieving. Many of those platitudes are religious. "God will never give us more than we can handle," can seem to mean "start handling this situation or it means that God lied." Or, "God needed another angel in heaven," can feel like, "God couldn't care less about your feelings, so he just *took* your child." Again, "God knows, even if we don't." This seems to mean that when we get to heaven God will have some kind of logical reason why Stephen died. I'm sorry to say it like this, but that's all bull shit. That's Patrick talking. Kristen doesn't say any bad words unless people are being mean to our kids. There's no good way to say this, but God refuses to give easy answers to complicated situations. When Job, a character in the Bible who had more grief than anyone should be forced to bear, spewed his anger at God, God did not explain himself. Interestingly, he just fought with Job. He matched Job's anger in an oddly satisfying way. One thing he did *not* say was, "Well, Job, here's the reason all your kids died and why I ruined your life." We believe God cares deeply for us when we are in grief. We believe that God understands the grief of losing a child because of Jesus' death on the Cross. After all, he was called the Son of God. God isn't often found in the platitude. More often God is found in the caring nurse, the supportive friend, the butterflies or birds, or poignant scripture verse or song that shows up at just the right time.

Churches can do better. Maybe that's an understatement. But after speaking to countless churches and church leaders, we *know* churches can do better. Many of them *are* doing wonderful things. Here are a few quick thoughts on how churches can serve moms and dads (or anyone else) in grief.

1. **Start a support group.** It could be seasonal, like eight weeks in the Spring. Or, it could be once a month, permanently. There are some great resources out there, like Resolve Through Sharing or GriefShare, that will help you develop the tools you need. All that is required is a space and time, and a leader with a heart for the hurting who understands how to create a safe space.

2. **Anniversary notes.** If you have a church office

of any kind, you can do this. Create a file system with a folder for each month of the year. If a person in the church has a loss during January, simply fill out a sympathy card and drop it in the "January" file. When January comes around the following year, pull out the note and drop it in the mail. You could also put the date on your digital calendar so you will be reminded when that time comes around.

3. **Training.** I speak to churches and church leaders on the topic of death, dying, grief, hospital visits, etc., often. A little training and candid conversation can go a long way.

4. **Special services.** Many churches host "Blue Christmas" services as a way to purposefully acknowledge those who have died and those who are in grief. Bereaved Mother's Day can also be a meaningful way to serve this population.

We could go on about this topic for a long time, but the bottom line is this. If you have been caught in some of the hurtful patterns of the church during your loss, we are so sorry. Churches need to do better. And they can do better.

21. When the Hospital Isn't Hospitable

Emmaline had a wonderful experience in the hospital. Lori just had an experience.

Let's face it, not many people apply for a job in a birthing center with the expectations that they will serve families at the *end* of life. They rightly anticipate serving them only at the *beginning* of life.

The hospital's strength is being safe and clinical. Not warm and fuzzy. Healthcare must be correct and appropriate, which isn't always the same as being caring and compassionate. Of course, all these attributes can and do often co-exist, but not always.

At our growing health system, Parkview Health, a system with nine hospitals and over 13,000 co-workers, every time a mom experiences a miscarriage or stillbirth, a chaplain is part of the team that responds. That means that at least one person will be coming from a softer standpoint. That chaplain will inform mom of her rights, give her grief information, and an invitation to support groups, send a sympathy card, maybe offer some memory-making, and generally care about the woman as a grieving mother. Mom will later be invited to a memorial service and have the chance for her baby's name to be read out loud as we light a candle and remember his or her brief life.

We wish we could say this was standard everywhere in the world. It most certainly is not.

Perhaps you would describe your experience of loss in a hospital (an emergency room, operating room, or birthing center) as cold and sterile instead of warm and caring.

Maybe you, like Lori, had clinical care that was fine and appropriate but didn't have much of a caring touch. Maybe you heard the words *fetal demise* and recoiled at the insensitivity as I did.

That's one of the reasons why I started Kindred Hearts. Kindred Hearts is a volunteer program that pairs a volunteer (or two) with every woman experiencing stillbirth in our two largest birthing centers. As we write this, I am coordinating

If you are connected to a health system that would like to learn more about what we have done at Parkview Health, please reach out to us through NoMatterHowSmallBook.com.

a response to support a mom whose baby, halfway through her second trimester, has died. These volunteers build on the excellent clinical care provided by our nurses. They focus on memory-making and the relational/emotional aspects of the patient. Since all of our volunteers have had a personal loss themselves, they approach the women with the kind of compassion that comes from personal experience.

If you are connected to a health system that would like to learn more about what we have done at Parkview Health, please reach out to us through NoMatterHowSmallBook.com.

If your loss experience at a hospital was less than caring, you're not alone, and we're so sorry. For many, this only adds to the pain of losing a child. It can add trauma to grief. We hope that every woman's experience is more like Emmaline's and less like Lori's.

22. Common Threads

Jayda, Emmaline, and Lori each had very different experiences. They each had different levels of support. As we conclude, let's consider some things they had in common.

1. **Their babies died.** That's obvious, but the problem with death is *permanence*. Whether your baby died when you were barely pregnant or was stillborn at full term, the pain you feel is because death separates us from those we love. That was the same for all three women.

2. **Hopes and expectations died, too.** Jayda and Toby were so excited to meet their brown-eyed baby girl. Emmaline worked so hard to create a family. Lori and the girls were already dressing Benjamin in cute little clothes in their imaginations. Each pregnancy brings with it thoughts of the future–hopes and expectations. When the pregnancy ends, those end, too.

3. **They all experienced grief.** Grief is caused by the absence of your child. Each mom lost something, *someone* they wanted. It has been said that *grief is love with no place to go.*

4. **Death came out of sequence.** Every parent expects to outlive their children. When Amani,

Baby Bethany, and Benjamin died, and their parents were still living, it felt so *wrong*. That's because it was. It's out of sequence. In those cases, parents were left behind by children.

5. **They are now part of a club no one wants to join.** I'm sure that all these parents would be happy to cancel their membership to the "loss parent" club if at all possible. However, there are certain benefits to being part of this club. We can appreciate our living children more if we are lucky enough to have them. We understand the pain of others a little better. I (Kristen) believe I am a better person because of my grief. I've met incredible people along this journey. I don't despise my grief any longer. It's my companion. It leads me and shapes me. I wish I didn't need it. But now that I have welcomed my grief, I notice the gifts that it has to offer.

In Conclusion

Thank you for picking up this book. We're not sure how you came across it, and we wish you didn't need it, but we hope it has helped you. We've given you:

- Practical resources
- Statistics and logistics about miscarriage and stillbirth
- Tools to honor and remember your baby that died
- Insight on facing grief and life after loss

Jayda and Toby, Emmaline, and Lori. These four people, and so many others embedded in their stories—Toby's dad, Jayda's mom, and sisters, Bethany, Emma, Jr., Micah and Haley, Jeff and Lori's girls, and Lori's counselor—leave an impression on our hearts. Why? Because stories of people facing miscarriage and stillbirth are profound and poignant. You've been there. So have we. You know. So do we.

Stories of grief and loss are never *happily ever after* stories. The pain of losing Stephen nearly 20 years ago is still with us. Our hearts still have cracks in them. But God has sprinkled good seeds in those heart-cracks. He's given us meaning and connection to him and others. We know Stephen is doing just fine. We won't pretend to know exactly what the afterlife looks like. But, when we sat alone together just after we learned that his heart stopped beating, I said to Patrick, "If you get there first, I'll be jealous. You'll get to see Stephen before me."

There is a joy set before us. That joy does not erase grief, but it does influence it. We will see Stephen again one day. Our arms will no longer be empty. We will know him completely and enjoy his presence. His absence will only be a memory. Until then, we believe he is in the arms of Jesus. If Stephen could not stay here with us, I am glad that he stays in the arms of our heavenly father. He skipped all the craziness and pain of living in this world and went right to eternity without tears, pain, or grief. We are confident we will be reunited.

Through Patrick's work at the hospital and my work with support groups, Kindred Hearts, and so many other opportunities, we work every day alongside moms and dads in deep grief over their lost children. Our hope for this book is that it joins us in the work we do, that it can be a place of support and refuge.

If we can serve you personally or an organization you care about, please go to NoMatterHowSmallBook.com, and click on the No Matter How Small page. Find us on Facebook and Instagram at "No Matter How Small Book". We'd love to connect with you.

One last thing. If you found this book helpful, would you please leave a review by clicking here or finding the book on Amazon? That would mean so much to us. It helps other people just like you meet Jayda, Emmaline, and Lori. Who knows? It could be just the resource they need in the middle of their grief. Please create a review now.

More Resources

Social Media

Patrick and I personally invite you to connect with the No Matter How Small community at "No Matter How Small Book" on Facebook or Instagram. Find encouragement, support, and connection to others who can sympathize with your grief journey. Follow "No Matter How Small Book" today.

Make an Impact on Your Group: Schedule a Live Presentation!

Has this book helped you? Do you know of a group that would benefit from a presentation of this content? Go to PatrickRiecke.com and book Kristen and Patrick Riecke to speak to your group today! Picture the concepts, education, and stories in this book, a life-changing conversation, and your group, better equipped than ever, to care for people experiencing this crisis. To schedule a keynote message, workshop, or event, go to PatrickRiecke.com now.

E-Mail Newsletter

While you are on the website, for more free content, videos, and advice on helping people who are sick, dying, or grieving, sign up for Patrick's free newsletter! When you sign up, you will receive access to many free tools and several video trainings where Patrick explains how to do what we have talked about in this book. Visit PatrickRiecke.com now to sign up.

Purchase the Other Books in the Series

If you found this book helpful, you might benefit from the rest of the series:

- *How to Talk with Sick, Dying, and Grieving People: When There are No Magic Words to Say* by Patrick Riecke
- *How to Find Meaning in Your Life Before it Ends* by Patrick Riecke
- *Giving a Life Meaning: How to Lead Funerals, Memorial Services, and Celebrations of Life* by Dr. Jon Swanson.

Wallet Cards for Hospital Visits

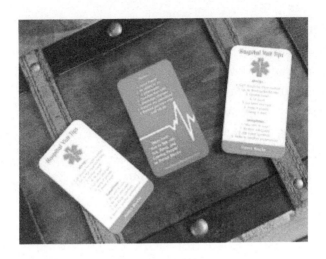

You never know when you will visit someone in a hospital. Be prepared with a FREE wallet card telling you what to ALWAYS, SOMETIMES, and NEVER do when you visit a hospital. Claim your wallet card today at PatrickRiecke.com/Resources.

Online Video Course

If this book was helpful, sign up for my (Patrick's) online video course today. Not only will you have access to video teaching based on my books, but you'll also learn:

- How to select a funeral home
- How to talk with children about death
- The difference between pain medication and assisted suicide
- How to perform advance care planning and find meaning in life

To begin my online video on demand course today, go to PatrickRiecke.com/courses.

Other Books in This Series

*How to Talk with Sick, Dying, and Grieving People:
When There are No Magic Words to Say*
by Patrick Riecke, 2018

How to Find Meaning in Your Life Before it Ends
by Patrick Riecke, 2019

*Giving a Life Meaning: How to Lead Funerals,
Memorial Services, and Celebrations of Life*
by Dr. Jon Swanson, 2020

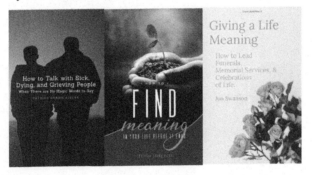

Thank You

The cover of *No Matter How Small* was created by a dear friend of ours, Tina Smith. The first time we saw it, we cried. The imagery is profound. After losing a baby, you may look the same from the outside, but something is missing. The wounds of grief are invisible but real. Like many people, Tina understands this experience firsthand, which is why she was able to graphically capture the feeling with the artwork on the front of this book. Thank you, Tina, for lending your talent and heart to this project.

A special thanks to our perennial proofreader, Nancy Swanson. Without her, commas would be, well, misplaced, everywhere. On a serious note, she excels in work few would be willing to do. She and Jon are special people who both understand the pain of a child's death firsthand, and spend professional energy helping grieving people. Thank you, Nancy. And, we're sorry that we skipped the classes that covered the proper use of a hyphen.

Acknowledgements

It's an honor to walk alongside those who experience stillbirth, miscarriage, and infant loss. We've had that honor in a wide variety of ways. Each of my (Kristen's) sisters and sisters-in-law have sadly had these experiences. My niece, Kamille (Kami) Jane Walls was born still at twenty-four weeks shortly after our daughter was born. I've had aunts and cousins share this experience, and even a toddler cousin, Kyle, who died when I was a young girl. Both of our mothers' first pregnancies ended in miscarriage. My grandmother, Loretta, delivered my twin uncles, James Ray and Joseph Roy in 1968. They both died shortly after birth, too small to survive. I grew up visiting their gravesite. Not long ago, Patrick's nephew, Zach, and his wife, Kelli, lost their daughter, Delaney Suzanne Bunn, on a day when we thought she would be born alive. Our family will never be the same. This book would not have been possible without so many family members sharing their hearts and grief with us.

As a teenager, I observed several influential people in my life as they went through the pain of miscarriage and stillbirth. My youth pastor and his wife, Bill and Trish O'Boyle, along with other families in my church (the Sextons and Hardins) all lost children while I was in high school. A close family friend, Andrea, who had been my babysitter when I was a child, experienced the devastating loss of her stillborn son, Alexander. Even as a young person, loss, and grief were **not** taboo. They were a part of my life in profound ways.

As adults, we have both watched many friends grieve as well. Dale and Sherry Gajewski walked this path many times, and let our hearts break with theirs each time. When we were newly married, our neighbors, Andy and Charla, gave birth to a stillborn baby girl. Later, they tenderly shared their feelings in the front room of our rented home. We lived across the street from the hospital where weeks later we would learn that our baby, Stephen, had died. After he died, friends comforted us. In many cases, we didn't even know they had losses until after our miscarriage. Among them were Kathy and Gary Martin, Nita Mousa, Randi Nussbaum, Cheri Dellinger, Kathy Klepper, and Cindy and Rob Shoaff.

In recent years, our lives have intersected with many more people who share this grief. We were very young when our miscarriage happened. As the years went on, many more friends had similar experiences. Additionally, through my work with support groups and the Kindred Hearts volunteer program, I have met some of the most compassionate and courageous people. We've served hundreds through these two programs, so it would be impossible to list them all, but here are a few special names of those people, and other friends with whom we have journeyed:

The Griesser family

The Ley family

The Kolkman family

Clayton Matthew Warren Thompson

Gavin Daniel 6/9/2015 and the Long family

Scott, Tanisha, Ainsley, Lochlan, and Cashel Faber

Chuck, Shelby and Charlie Zook

The Ross family

Avery Elizabeth Rife, 11/24/2011-11/25/2011 and family

Ella, Jack, Benjamin, and the Bernard family

Gabriel Thomas Larmondra and family

Madilyn Corine Alejandro

Justin, Justine, William, Nessa, and Lilly Shirley

Joe, Mackenzie and Baby Theodore

Lisa Marie Phillips and my "Blueberry" babies

Cole, Abby, Everleigh, & Aurora "Rory" Irene Applegate

The Holler family, Josh Leslie, Landon, Sloane, and Cole

The Hartleib family

Morgan Lynn and the Johns family

The Weiland family

The Kirk family

Jennifer, Brandon, Emerie 8/4/2016-8/7/2016, Elie 3/9/2017, and Aria

Kody, Tessa and Kolt Lee Jackson

Scott, Nikki, and Baby Madison Rose Gase

Marc, Delaney, and Rowan Joy Baumann

The Barney family

Justin, Deidre and Abram Levi

The Babbitt family

Abigail Skye, Noel, and the DuMond family

Oliver 6/27/2016-7/5/2016 and Stephen, Danielle, Atticus, Jordyn, Braxton, Camden, and Felicity Bush

Natalee Marie Umberg and family

And, most especially, Tim, Cori, Claire, Norah, & June McKenzie

We hold a special appreciation for these people who support loss families in our area:

Barb Kramer, RN

Melinda Leatherman, RN

Kristin Koning, *Noah's Bears*

Michelle Glenn, *Loving Benjamin*

Jennifer Potter and Jessi Snapp, *Now I Lay Me Down to Sleep*

The Baumann family, *Remembering Rowan*

Julie Lehman, *Hope Mommies*

Made in the USA
Coppell, TX
12 January 2021